Ambulance!

Real Stories from a Small-Town ER

Kerry Hamm

Disclaimer:

Names, locations, and portions of the details included in this book have been altered to protect the privacy of those involved.

If you haven't read the first three books, don't worry. Let me fill you in on a few things:

Welcome to a small-town Emergency Room in Ohio. With six trauma bays, one mental health room, one low pressure room, one quarantine room, and 11 other exam bays, this ER has the capacity to fit 21 patients at a time, with more than 100 patients often lining up in the lobby and waiting room on any given evening shift.

We're no big-shot inner city hospital. We transfer out burns and severe pediatric cases. We have a mental health floor, inpatient rehab, intermediate care/critical care, and hospice floor in addition to pediatrics, general surgery, obstetrics, and nursery floors. Unless patients are directly admitted from facilities in surrounding areas, they show up in our department first.

My name is Kerry and I'm the first person you'll see when you come through those ER doors: registration. Now, it seems a lot of people wouldn't mind to hear the following stories (or previous) if they came from the patient's doctor(s) or nurse(s), but there seems to be some kind of 'offensive' nature if the stories come from registration. I'm going to put that to rest and say I love my job, I love being the first staff member to interact with all of these patients, and I try my best to treat every patient with the utmost respect.

On any given day, two to three clerks work during the day and evening shifts, taking turns gathering names, birth dates, and diagnoses at the front (while juggling floor transfers, admits from surrounding hospitals, and outside phone calls from some cat lady named Linda who's making her third call this shift to see if we think she needs to come in for tingling in her left butt cheek), and then in the back, where we enter patients' rooms to gather contact and insurance information to complete the registration process.

It used to be, once 11 p.m. hit, I waved to my coworkers as they walked out the door, and I was left at the registration desk with a triage nurse in a small room behind the desk, security lurking behind a two-way mirror that takes up an entire wall in front of the registration desk, a not-so-empty waiting room to my right, and six registered nurses and one or two doctors in the back.

Well, it turns out someone was paying attention, so a few days out of my week-long stretches, I have an awesome coworker at my side for a couple of hours.

When I first started the first book, I didn't think there would be a second. And then, the third was going to be 'the very last.' But then all hell broke loose one night, and I realized there's never going to be a shortage of stories.

Almost story here is true (see the next paragraph), though dialogue has been changed slightly, all names have been changed, and some situations have been slightly altered to protect patient privacy. It has never been my intention to exploit the heartaches or embarrassments of others,

2

but simply offer a glimpse into the world of the Emergency Room, where every patient seems to be a wild card.

I decided to have a little bit of fun with this book. Four of the stories included here never happened...at least not at this hospital. Which stories are just too crazy to be true? The answers are located near the end of the book.

An After-Christmas Story

There are several things I enjoy hearing if I'm being woken by a phone call. These are as follows:

"Hey, you've won the lottery!"

"Hey, I've won the lottery, and I want to give you half of it!"

"I brought you food."

"We're still going to pay you, but you don't need to come to work tonight."

Okay, I've actually never heard any of those things upon answering the phone out of a dead sleep, but when my phone rang on my day off, three hours in my sleep schedule, I would have rather heard one of the previous.

Boy, I can't get lucky.

"Hey, so [the hospital 30 minutes away, the only other hospital within an hour of us] went up in flames. They're sending all of their patients here. We need help."

I could have lied. I could have said I was drunk or

hungover. I could have told the truth and explained I'd been fighting a wicked ear infection and cold all weekend. Or I could have just said what I was thinking: it's my last day off before I have to work another seven in a row, and I really don't feel like coming in tonight.

Did I say any of those things? Of course not.

"Let me get dressed," I said. "I'll be in as soon as my car warms up."

I scrambled to get ready, knowing I was about to jump into a disaster.

And then I went outside.

"What the fudge?"

Come on, get real. I don't say fudge. You know what I said when I saw another four inches of snow had fallen over the five that fell that morning.

I looked out to the road in front of my house. There were a few swervy tire tracks, but other than that, the road hadn't been plowed. The snow had drifted and almost reached the top of my tires.

"You're kidding me," I sighed.

After getting my car windows scraped off, getting the car defrosted, and popping my beat-up SUV in 4WD just to get out of the driveway, I headed to work.

Let me gripe for a minute.

I don't know about your hospital, but at this one—and leading to it—the roads are never clear in winter. Now, if you need liquor or pizza, rest assured you'll get to those stores just fine, since the paths to those places are always clear. But if you need to, I don't know, drive really fast to the emergency room because you just cut your toe off while you were trying to channel Bill Murray in *Groundhog Day* and use a chainsaw to carve an angel in an ice block (which is a real story, but that's about it in a nutshell), forget about going over 10 MPH, and then press your luck once you pull in the hospital parking lot.

Seriously, we have some periods of time when our patients aren't from out in town, but coworkers checking in because they busted their butts trying to leave or come inside.

My walk through the parking lot and into the ER took about 10 times the length of that rant.

And as soon as I walked in, I wanted to walk out.

I contemplated it.

None of my coworkers had noticed me yet. Not one of the 9000 people in the waiting room or lobby paid me a lick of attention. I kept telling myself I could just leave and nobody would ever be the wiser.

But dang it, I'm a good person.

You already have the impression that it was busy, and it was. I took a look at the Tracking Board, and all but one of the patients were checked in for serious chief complaints, such as chest pain or lacerations that required transfers.

Our phones rang off the hook. My coworkers were scrambling to keep paperwork organized, while they took transfer and floor admit orders and simultaneously registered the never-ending sea of people in the lobby.

Someone handed me a stack of papers.

"These are all the people from that other hospital. The floors are saying they need us to call that place and see if we can get medical records."

While I worked on that, calling the up-in-flames facility and every other hospital within two hours, trying to get our patients' records, the Tracking Board filled up. At one point, there were too many ambulances in the bay to hold one more. So then EMS began parking in front of the ER entrance and wheeled stretchers in through the lobby. The people waiting spread like the Red Sea. Granted, it did take a few "Get out of my way, now"s to get the people moved...

"Turn on the scanner so we know what's coming in," I instructed one of my coworkers.

She turned on security's police scanner, and we caught the tail end of a conversation. The dispatcher said a patient was coming by car because of the wait time for an ambulance. I thought it sounded like the dispatcher was laughing, but I brushed it off.

Because we weren't busy enough and I sometimes can't stop myself from saying aloud what I'm thinking, I ticked off my coworkers by announcing cheerfully, "Well, at least [name of an obnoxious, drug addicted, violent frequent flyer] isn't here tonight."

Nobody even had time to groan before that man entered the ER.

The man cut to the front of the line. I was pre-admitting an account, and my coworker was helping another patient register.

"Sign me in so I don't have to wait," he barked at me.

"Sir," I sternly replied, "you know that's not how it works. Unless you are at death's door right now, you'll have to wait in line like everyone else."

He was fuming.

"My girlfriend's sister came over tonight and took all of my hydros. I've been going to three hospitals to get those. Sign me in so I can get more."

I once again explained to the man that he'd have to wait like everyone else.

And that's when he took the bottle of hand sanitizer from the counter, chucked it toward the waiting room windows, and watched as the impact shattered the glass.

(That's not how you use that!)

Some of the people in the waiting room screamed. Some of the people in the lobby screamed. A few people from both areas excused themselves and left the building. Nobody, however, felt it either safe or their responsibility to become involved with the situation.

If there had ever been a time to use the hidden-under-the-counter emergency button to alert security, it was right then.

"Sign me in," the guy yelled at me.

I ignored three direct admit calls as I tried to keep the patient calm by complying to his demand.

During the registration process, I kept wondering where security was.

Then I heard a woman from the back shout out every obscenity I've heard of, some that I'm sure came straight out of 1837, and there was possibly a bit of

Klingon in there as well. (No joke...when I came home later, I had to Google one of the words: bescumber. By the way, if you don't know what that is, don't Google it at work.) That took care of trying to track down the location of security.

I finished registering the man and tried to direct him to the waiting room, but that worked about as well as trying to explain to him the first time around that he needed to wait in line.

He spit on me and I wanted to retaliate, but I also wanted to keep my job and kept telling myself that the patient was probably under the influence or in the desperate stages of withdrawal.

"Let me just call the back and find out where they want you, okay?" I said, as I wiped the man's bodily fluid from my right cheek.

I went to the back office and called 911.

"An officer is about a half block from you," the dispatcher said. "Can you wait that long?"

I responded that I would try to stall the man.

"Does he have a weapon?" asked the dispatcher.

I told the woman on the other line about the waiting room window. She said she would send another unit in addition to the nearest, and she asked if I could move the patient away from other patients and visitors.

"Sir," I said, as I returned to the lobby, "we're going to move you to a special room."

Can you believe that this caused an uproar among the patients in the lobby and those who'd walked out of the waiting room to get a better glimpse of all the action?

"I have been here for three hours already," shrieked a woman. She was holding a newborn and pacing the hallway. When she yelled, the baby woke up and followed her cue to wail.

She continued, "My husband's sister works here. You need to see employees and family of employees first."

"I have to be at work in the morning," another patient chimed in. "I can't go in, coughing like this. Do I need to break a window, too?"

"Shut your faces," said our drug seeker. "I'm going to a special room. Didn't ya'll hear the lady?"

As I walked the man to a room we only use to store old waiting room chairs, I think just about every person I passed called me a curse word. I really wanted to turn around and explain to these people that I was doing the best I could to keep them safe, but I'm sure that would have been met with the same warmth.

I left the man in the chair room with assurance that the room was a 'fast track' room (one meant for in and out patients or for patients without traumatic injuries or diagnosing complications) and went back to the registration desk.

My coworkers were directing four cops to the chair room. Two of the officers drew their weapons. I prayed the man in the room didn't have a weapon, and I prayed the officers would not have to resort to using their firearms.

As the officers walked away from the registration guest, a sobbing college student walked inside. Her six friends surrounded her.

"What's going on?" I questioned the crying girl.

She kept sobbing and didn't make an attempt to answer the question.

I turned to her friends.

"Guys, can you tell me why she's here tonight?"

One of the girls in the group snickered.

"Remember that movie they play over and over and over again on Christmas?"

"*A Christmas Story?*" I asked.

The same girl nodded and held her hands over her mouth to stifle her laughter.

"You didn't shoot your eye out, did you?" I joked, hoping to lighten the situation.

The sobbing girl shook her head.

I tried to think of my favorite parts of that movie to narrow down the list of what could be wrong with the girl.

There went the screaming and physical altercation between the cops and the drug seeker down the hall.

"She's an idiot," one of the girl's friends said.

She nudged the girl. "Open your mouth and show her."

Yeah. Then I remembered that scene.

"Seriously?" I asked, with big, wide eyes.

The girl slowly stuck out her tongue. The tip was gone.

Police officers were still fighting the man down the hall.

"She stuck her tongue to the pole and it froze," one of the girl's friends said. "We didn't even know it'd really work, but it did."

Of course it did. It was like two degrees outside.

"You didn't use warm water to loosen the adhesion?"

All of the college kids looked at each other like, 'We could have done THAT? Why didn't we do that?'

Instead, I guess they opted to...

Wait for it.

As I was writing this, I just had to take a huge breath and sigh because I still can't believe someone could be so dumb...six times over.

Instead of pouring water over the girl's tongue, her friends got the bright idea to go the *Sixteen Candles* direction—you know, the part where someone could have just opened the bedroom door to get Caroline's hair unstuck— and they cut the tip of the girl's tongue off by using a pair of scissors.

They cut off part of her freaking tongue!

"She just needs to get it looked at and know when it's going to grow back."

What are you, a lizard?

"Ummmm..."

By now, the cops were dragging the pill guy out the front doors and I was trying to get the tongue patient registered.

As far as I know, our hydro guy is still in jail. I guess he had a few warrants out for his arrest.

And the tongue girl...She learned her severed tongue would heal, but it wouldn't grow back. I think she's probably still trying to get used to living a life with a square-tipped tongue.

Giving Children Their Wings

Our frequent flyers aren't always adults. Some of our frequent patients are children with chronic health issues, such as asthma, CHF, cancer, and even mental health.

Here are two stories about the latter.

During the month of December, most parents are scrambling from store to store, purchasing those items their children 'just have to' have, and spend countless hours after the kids go to bed just to wrap those gifts and stick them under the tree. And it's a great feeling, right, to see those little eyes widen and sparkle?

For some, Christmas season doesn't go so well.

That was the case for one of our frequent flyers, a young girl diagnosed with a mental health disorder where she was defiant against authority. After years of her parents admitting they 'never dared' tell her the word 'no,' mom and dad felt that was catching up to them, and they decided to (finally) take medical advice to enter a family therapy program. We hadn't seen the family for some time, so we figured the program was working for them.

We learned that it wasn't when a call came over that the patient stabbed her mother.

This child, not even in her teen years, *stabbed* her mother with a steak knife.

Our child patient was brought in via ambulance, restrained to her gurney with black canvas ties. She

14

was screaming at the top of her lungs and I'm pretty sure I heard words come out of her mouth that I didn't use well until I was in my adult years.

The patient was placed in our monitored mental health room, and our mental health counselor was called in to try to calm the patient.

Multiple nurses attempted to calm the patient verbally, with the threat of sedative a last resort. The patient refused to comply and chewed at her restraints and through two IV tubes. She also voided her bowels and repeatedly held her breath until she nearly passed out.

Finally, our mental health counselor arrived.

Her first order of business was speaking to the patient's parents to learn what brought on the behavior the family had been working to correct.

Get ready.

Are you ready?

Our frequent flyer stabbed her mother because she was told she could only open two presents per night, leading up to Christmas morning. The patient had already opened two presents that night, but the child demanded she be allowed to open the remaining 30-something gifts under the tree.

According to mom, the patient threw her 'typical' tantrum: the child tossed things about, threw the television remote at the television (and broke the screen), and kicked her.

Mom said she prided herself in diffusing the situation. She then sent her child to time out.

While mom was trying to pick up the glass from the broken television, the patient took a secret trip to the kitchen, grabbed a knife from the knife block, and unsuspectingly stabbed her mother in the lower back.

Our mental health counselor urged the patient's mother to register as a patient herself, to which she complied. (She ended up getting something like 14 stitches.)

Throughout the child's stay in the ER, she cursed, bit, kicked, and spit at nurses and staff. She was eventually transferred to another hospital equipped to treat minors with mental health disorders.

Our second child came to visit us a few days after the holidays, when he apparently was still fuming that he didn't get what he wanted for Christmas.

Now, with this patient, you already know more than I did when my coworker was registering him.

During the time the patient was at the desk, I was running back and forth to the unit clerk, delivering paperwork and trying to catch up on charts. So when I went back up to the desk, just as the patient's registering process was wrapping up, I didn't think much about the pre-teen boy missing his shirt. See, patients sometimes disrobe right there at the counter because they think registration needs to see that 'rash' or boil on a penis or 'radioactive spider bite.' (We don't.)

My coworker asked our patient's mother to head on over to the waiting room, but mom didn't listen. She said she'd rather stand by the ER doors.

Okay, whatever.

My coworker went to the back for a minute, and I continued registering another patient and his companion at the desk. It was busy, and I never stopped to look at the diagnosis for the previous patient. I didn't hear anyone screaming or fighting or doing anything out of the ordinary, and I couldn't see where the previous family stood, so, you know, I minded my own business and tried to do my job.

Before I knew it, the patient at the desk became distracted and started nervously glancing toward the door.

Our security guards rushed to the lobby and bombarded the triage nurse.

"This boy needs a room now," they kept telling the confused nurse.

The next thing I knew, someone was rushing to the lobby with a gown.

Okay. I had to stand up and find out what was going on.

Whew.

There was our patient, fully undressed, urinating all over the lobby floor while everyone and their brothers watched.

And what were the parents doing? Mom was covering her face. Dad was laughing.

A tech ran to the lobby and tried to wrap a blanket around the patient, but the child refused. Finally, the tech stopped asking and wrapped the blanket around the kid. Our tech politely asked the child to follow him, but the kid didn't want anything to do with compliance. Again, our tech stopped asking and carried the child back to a stat-cleaned room.

Well, we started thinking everything would be okay. Housekeeping was called to clean up the urine. Our charge nurse called in a mental health counselor. We didn't hear screaming from the back...

So we just kept working.

We kept working until we saw security bolt from the room around the same time four city police officers ran inside.

There I was, thinking maybe another ETOH patient was brought in or something.

Nope.

Our naked boy from earlier was destroying his room, so much so that security was bypassed and city officers were called in. The boy somehow managed to loosen and remove the faucet from the in-room sink, tear a hole in his cot, shred sheets, smash a chair over the counter, hit two nurses, and bite a tech so hard the patient's tooth broke off and the tech had to get stitches.

From nurse reports, dad found all of this hilarious. He was asked to leave the patient's room.

While mental health tried to find a place to take the patient, we learned the parents brought the child to the ER because he was 'out of control' at home. Right before coming to the ER, he pushed over the Christmas tree, busted out two living room windows, took a pair of scissors to the bathroom wall, and set his bedroom carpet on fire.

Our people called around for hours, trying to find a transfer facility, but for one reason or another, nobody would take the patient.

Finally, eight hours and FOUR sedation shots later, our patient was transferred out.

We haven't heard anything about the second patient, but we learned our first patient has resumed family therapy sessions.

And yes, we've all wondered what's going to happen when these kids are teenagers and adults. You're not alone.

I Know That's Not Why You're Here, But...

To be completely honest, I have debated heavily about putting this story in any of my books because I still can't explain how I feel about it, even after a great deal of time has passed.

Most people come to the ER because they don't want to die. Okay, that's what the ER was made for, but I'm not so sure anymore that's the primary reason patients come to see us. Still, the purpose of the emergency room is to create an environment suitable for the best healthcare professionals to offer assistance in keeping a patient alive.

One family had a different idea.

An elderly man was brought in via ambulance. Nobody knew too much about the patient, other than it was called over the radio that the man was foaming at the mouth and coding. He was well beyond his 80s, and he was living at an assisted living facility after the death of his wife.

It didn't sound like anything I haven't seen before. Nurses were readying a room, and the only doctor on shift was barking orders at everyone in sight.

Then the patient was wheeled down the hall by EMS.

I went back to the registration desk, wondering if the patient's family or friends would show up.

And they did.

All 25 of them.

Surprisingly, the family already designated a spokesperson: the patient's grandson.

"Is he dead?" the man asked.

I shook my head. "For now, he's still alive. But they are working on him, and they're going to need a little bit of time before I can send anyone back to see him."

My answer didn't please the family. Several of the man's grandchildren and great-grandchildren groaned and walked off.

"I'm sorry," I said, thinking the family groaned because I couldn't send anyone back to visit, "but they just need a little bit of time to get him stabilized."

The grandson shook his head.

"It's not that," he replied. "Look, can I talk to a nurse or a doctor? This is important."

I called to the back and asked the unit clerk to notify one of the patient's nurses about the family's request. I was told everyone was busy, so it would be a few minutes.

"I don't have a few minutes," the grandson grunted to me, after I relayed the message. "I need to talk to someone now."

I went to the back and got my head bitten off as I informed the room full of nurses and the doctor of the grandson's beckoning.

The doctor yelled, "Will someone just go and find out what the family wants?"

A flustered RN, new to the unit at the time, walked to the front with me. She introduced herself to the grandson, and as soon as the rest of the family noticed there was a nurse out front, they gathered around.

"We're doing everything we can to save your grandfather," the nurse told the patient's grandson.

He scowled. "That's what I'm afraid of."

The nurse was confused. "Excuse me?"

A woman from the group explained, "This is his sixth suicide attempt this year. Every single time he tries to die and fails, he gets meaner. He hates his life. He tells us all the time he hates us for not killing him."

"Yeah," another woman chimed in. "My husband and I moved him in with us after grandma died, but then my eight-year-old caught grandpa sprinkling rat poison on oatmeal. Can you imagine, hearing from your daughter at the crack of dawn that your grandpa's trying to kill himself in your kitchen? He was in Critical Care for two months. We had to take him to a home after that. I can't have that around my kid. And I can't watch him twenty-four-seven."

The nurse and I probably had the same looks on our faces. I know my eyes were frozen in a widened position, but when I realized my reaction, I tried to blink 800 times and twitch my nose to get my facial expression to go back to normal.

"You have to either let him die," the grandson pleaded, "or you have to kill him."

"Sir," the nurse stated, "what you're telling me concerns me. I'm going to have to report this to social services."

The man shrugged. "We've been reported before. Look, I know it sounds like we're these horrible people, asking you to kill our relative, but every time he fails, he comes back and gets more creative. And he's just mean. He used to be so nice, but now all he does is yell and blame us for not letting him die. Please. Please, just let him die. He's going to be so mad if he lives again."

The nurse went to the back to report all of this to the ER doctor. During this time, I guess the nursing home called and said they found empty medication bottles in the patient's dresser drawers. None of the medications were prescribed to him, but to other nursing home residents. The patient apparently played poker for medication and stole pills from other residents' rooms. He then emptied all the pill bottles into a rag, took the pills, and overdosed with the rag still in his hand.

The patient did die.

His family actually cried and thanked the nurses for letting the man die, but none of the nurses had much to do with it. There were no advance directives in place, so the goal was to save the patient. It just so happened nature had other plans.

Someone in the family suggested they go out for dinner to celebrate, and they started making plans to have a 'death party' instead. I still am not over the shock of hearing family members talk about splitting the price of a keg three-ways and try to negotiate who was bringing what food directly after a patient's death, despite the length of time that has passed since this incident.

The grandson came in a few months later and gave us an update. Apparently, the patient's toxicology report showed the man ingested critical levels of Actonel, Coumadin, Lotensin, Desyrel, and more than 10 other medications that I couldn't remember.

<u>Give and Take</u>

There's a lot of balance in the ER. I won't call it karmic balance because I can't understand why a 40-something-year-old chronic polysubstance abuser/rapist/convicted murderer lives, yet a two-month-old dies after the first patient ran a red light while high on drugs.

But we see a lot of senseless give and take...Call me negative, I guess, but I see the take a lot more than I see the give. One patient will probably never know the life that was taken the night she was given hers.

Our night wasn't coming along too badly. After a long week of getting slammed, patients were coming in sporadically and for petty complaints, such as back pain or superficial lacerations that required little more than a bandage or a single stitch.

We were sitting around the desk, listening to security's police scanner.

"Be advised we received a call regarding a female subject, age in the late twenties or thirties. Her roommate called and said he walked in on the subject trying to hang herself. The beam gave and the patient fell. Now the roommate is telling us the subject left the house and may be a danger to herself. It is unclear at this time if the subject is a danger to others, so operate on the assumption that she is until you can assess."

It wasn't a shock. Around the holidays, we hear lots of calls like that.

Around the same time, an ambulance came in hot with a girl under the age of two. She was thought to be experiencing an allergic reaction. The patient was experiencing shortness of breath, was broken out in a rash, and was thought to be running a fever—which actually turned out to be a fever of 105-something-degrees.

Mom and dad accompanied the child, and both came out periodically to answer registration questions or call family.

Then the nurses locked down the back. Nobody goes in. Nobody comes out. We knew someone's health had taken a turn for the worst. We don't lock down our ER like that unless every nurse and doctor are needed in one room.

That baby hadn't cried in a minute and a half. We heard mom crying loudly from the hall.

It wasn't hard to figure out which room all our people were in.

Then another call came over the police scanner.

"Subject has been located. She's standing on the bridge, crying."

We listened to the cops talking about trying to coax the woman down from the bridge. It seemed to go on forever, but I don't think more than a few minutes had passed.

And then something amazing happened.

The woman slipped on a patch of ice and fell—

backwards.

An ambulance brought the woman in for a head injury with no open wound and a mental eval.

Meanwhile, that toddler in the other room still wasn't doing much better. When I walked by, the child was lifeless. I heard nurses yelling to one another that her respiratory responses sped up rapidly, while her blood pressure dropped. Lab couldn't draw samples. Her skin was speckled with a nasty rash that covered her entire body.

Mom and dad did their best to soothe the child, to let her know they were still by her side.

Our suicide attempt was lucky. She didn't even have a concussion, and she said she thought she would be okay eventually, but she was just upset that her boyfriend (a.k.a. 'roommate') had just broken up with her.

As she was being discharged, right at the moment that word showed up on the tracking board, the child in the other room died.

It wasn't an easy night. It's never easy for any of us when something like this happens. Nurses and doctors did everything within their power to keep that child alive, yet some stronger 'power' was pulling her away. We watched the parents and family go back and forth between the consult rooms and the patient's room, sobbing.

I try not to think too much about the give and take we see around here, but there are times I wish people understood a little more why we all say we love and hate our jobs in the ER.

27

Every now and then, I can't help but ask "Seriously?" to a registering patient's chief complaint. I very rarely use it to reference the actual complaint, but that the patient thinks it warrants a trip to the emergency room.

The latest complaint to illicit this response?

"I was punched in the elbow four days ago."

<u>Stalkers Aren't Born, They're Made</u>

If you read this story, you'll hopefully understand instantly why I don't consider it funny in the slightest. I've spoken to coworkers and have discovered just about every single female working in our department has experienced something similar during her career.

I'm pretty sure I've talked about my 'luck' in the other books. When I say I have 'luck,' what I really mean is I have the *wonderful pleasure* of experiencing some of the finer things in life, like disasters that occur with a two-percent chance of it happening to someone, getting stopped by every train in town, only to also get stopped by every red light, and then I get to work and learn that wasn't even the bad part: we're also super busy and all of my clocks were somehow set an hour behind, so now I'm late for work and everyone's mad.

Oh, and I have another 'lucky' trait: I attract creepy men. And when I say creepy, I mean...men like this next patient.

I first met this man on my first day off of a long-awaited three-day weekend. After clocking out, I headed straight to the store to stock up on cleaning supplies. (Yes, my life is so exciting that I spend a full day catching up on laundry, dishes, scrubbing the tub, and mopping.)

Upon checkout, my cashier noted my cleaning supplies and I (stupidly) told him I had three-days of cleaning to do. And then he started hitting on me. I didn't think much of it, and I tried my best to be polite, though I did explain I wasn't interested.

The cashier then saw the name badge I hardly ever wear (for this exact purpose) clipped to my jacket. He asked a few questions about work, and then he wanted to escort me to my car to help with my bags.

I declined that offer, given I only had two bags and a new broom, but the cashier insisted. Finally, to my surprise and great relief, his coworker stepped in and told him, essentially, to leave me alone because it was clear I was not interested and I appeared 'creeped out.'

That was a good term to use, and as things progressed, it turned out to be truer than I ever imagined.

On my first night back, I walked in and noticed a few people on the Tracking Board. We weren't incredibly busy, but I thought I would give my coworkers a break from the back, so I printed out a few face sheets and went to finish registering patients.

Wouldn't you know, the very first room I entered held the cashier from a few days earlier?

Hey, it's a small town. These things happen.

"I've been wanting to see you," he said.

These things apparently happen, too.

I saw the patient's complaint was for alcohol dependency.

While I was in the room, I tried to remain

professional. Usually, I can be in and out of a room in no time at all, but this man was a brand new patient, so none of his information was on file. During the time I tried to get the information, at least five 'will you go out with me' questions were thrown in between my questions of his address and contact information.

Finally, and I mean FINALLY, I gathered my information, told the man I wasn't interested and definitely don't date patients, and I left the room.

This didn't deter the man.

Promptly upon discharge, he approached the registration desk and talked and talked and talked some more. Nothing I could do or say would make him leave me alone. But like a check for a million dollars that comes when you're broke and tired of eating Ramen for two years straight, another miracle happened: his ride, an ambulance service car, arrived. I mouthed a thank you to the sky as the man left.

Well, none of this has been the creepy part.

See, the man kept coming to the ER. In a month, he graced me with his presence 16 times. Two more times, he showed up at work, but I wasn't there, so he was an LBT (left before triage). It got to the point that the man called before coming in, and he recognized my voice over the phone, even when I took to using a fake name when I answered outside calls. Each time he would come in, he tried to talk to me at the desk, in the hall, in his room...anywhere he could. Security and other staff members took great care of me once I explained the situation.

The man mostly came in for alcoholic issues or

mental health. At times, his BAC would be .58. No matter how much he stumbled around when he would get out of bed to try to find me, and no matter what seemed to be ailing him, he would come up with an excuse to try to speak with me.

One night, after his 'normal' visit didn't pan out the way he wanted it to, the man took to illegal consumption of toxic products…spray paint, okay? The man bought spray paint and started huffing it. He then called the cops on himself, continued huffing in front of officers, and dared them to take him to jail. But due to the man's alcohol intoxication, he had to be brought in for medical clearance. And he knew what he was doing because the cops explained the man knew it was a sure way to get back to the ER.

Hey, I said he was creepy, not stupid.

Well, maybe he's a bit stupid, too.

While the patient was awaiting clearance to be carted off to jail, he saw me in the back and started flailing his arms.

The man tried to get out of bed, but when his feet touched the floor, I guess the level of alcohol and fumes in his system hit him all at once because he fell face down to the floor. Nurses ran to make sure the patient didn't hurt himself, but he wasn't worried about that at all.

"Hey," he yelled, as nurses helped him back to bed. "Come here. I didn't get to talk to you earlier, so I came back."

I ignored him.

"Come on in here. I need you."

33

I finally looked the man in the eye from my spot in the nurse's station and said, "I don't want to talk to you. I'm not coming in there."

I then asked the man's arresting officer to sign consent, and I started to walk away.

Distraught over the rejection, the patient began slamming his head against the bed railing. He then got on his knees, turned around, and started slamming his head against the wall.

"I'm going to kill myself, you know," he screamed. "Come talk to me."

The man was taken to jail shortly after the incident.

I discussed the gentleman with a police officer. Legally, the man's trips to the ER could be considered 'coincidental' to my work schedule, especially given I work a week or more at a time. As long as the man was coming in for medical treatment and was not harassing me outside of work, I could not take legal action. The officer advised me to speak with the mental health unit to notify them of the patient's behavior, as well as discuss the incidents with security. I then learned the patient was registered as a violent sex offender.

None of this was making me feel safer.

Then I started finding gifts on my porch at home. The first package was a small box that was left a few days after a family friend left gifts while I was sleeping, so I figured the box was from someone who knew my schedule and knew not to knock. The gift was a little weird to me…it was a jewel-studded choker necklace. I don't really wear jewelry, but I thought maybe a friend thought I didn't wear any because I didn't own any.

Okay. It was a nice gesture.

But then other gifts started popping up. Someone was leaving clothes, desserts, jewelry, blankets...I asked around at work and every person I knew outside of work. Nobody fessed up to the gifts, and I started becoming paranoid, but one of my friends at work suggested maybe a coworker left the gifts because they wanted to help me out, but they didn't want me to feel obligated to return the favor. So I thought that meant she may have left the gifts, and I suddenly felt that maybe I would offend her if I didn't use some of the gifts.

I wore one of the blouses left gift-wrapped on my porch to work one night, and I ran into the man again.

"Nice shirt," he called out to me as I passed his room. "I bet you really like that color, right? And isn't it soft?"

My heart stopped and I almost threw up.

The man wouldn't confess to leaving the gifts at my house, and when I talked to officers, they said without proof that the man left the boxes, I couldn't really do anything about it. An officer volunteered to patrol my street for a few days, but nothing ever came of it.

Now, I've always been the type to make sure cars weren't following me home after work, but my paranoia started getting out of control. I was afraid to go out to my car when I realized I left a drink in it, scared to death that the man would be in my yard. I made my dog walk with me everywhere, even to the bathroom or to change laundry from the washer to the dryer. And I avoided going out. I avoided the store the man worked at, avoided the stores around it, and avoided going to public places, such as fast food restaurants, all in fear he would be there. In a tiny town, that's not an easy task. I started having nightmares of the patient finding my house, breaking in, and trying to kill me. The dreams were so vivid that I wouldn't be able to go back to sleep. I paid closer attention to even the slightest shadow in the parking lot as I was coming to and leaving work. And on my shifts, every time that police scanner went off, a pit grew in my stomach that it'd be the man.

During one of my week-long stretches, the man came in every single day, sometimes twice during my shifts.

The last time I saw the man (two nights ago), he was brought in via ambulance. When I learned he was four times the legal limit with alcohol intoxication, I skipped the consent form with a loophole that the patient was ETOH and his signature wouldn't be admissible. Since he'd only been in there a thousand times recently, I filed through his chart. I did this so I wouldn't have to interact with him.

He was discharged and security made sure to sit at the desk with me while the patient carried around a frozen TV dinner someone from the back gave him just to get him to go home.

The guard's presence didn't deter the man from trying to talk to me, but I guess someone called the cops and they came in just in the nick of time.

"Sir, why did you call 911 tonight?" asked one of the officers.

He shrugged. "I needed help."

"Did you have a medical emergency?"

The man froze.

The cop looked at the TV dinner. "Were you just hungry?"

"No," said the man with a laugh. "I just..."

"Were you bleeding? Were you experiencing a life or death situation?"

The man stammered through a bunch of incoherent gibberish.

"You've called 911 three times this week for transport. You do understand 911 is for life-threatening emergencies only, right? It wasn't designed to be a taxi."

The patient looked at me and tried to speak.

"I suggest you go home and think about why you felt the need to dial 911," the cop said, cutting the man off. "And if you call 911 again without experiencing a life-threatening emergency, I will take you to jail."

I'm updating this right as I'm finishing this book for release. You know, I want to say there was a good ending to this, but it's still ongoing.

The patient has eased up on bothering me as much, but it's still an issue if he can catch me when I'm alone at the desk or if I have to enter his room for any reason.

He was arrested a few times since the TV dinner night, but each time was bailed out.

He's threatened suicide a few times, each when I refused to communicate with him.

A Hot Family Affair

It was about three in the morning, on my night off, no less, when I heard the police scanner go off. I wasn't going to pause my movie and get out of my pajamas for one ambulance alert, but when I saw a bunch of cops and firetrucks speed by my house, I paid a little more attention to the radio.

According to dispatchers, a house located across town was on fire and several residents were trapped inside.

We all know that's no good. And, well, I worried about my coworker because when you're working alone, just two or three patients at once can become a mess. Add on families, friends, and emergency responders and... well, it makes you stop and wonder what you ever did to deserve to be in such hell.

When emergency responders stated they were told there were six people (one adult and five children) trapped in one upstairs room of the house, I figured that was a good indication that I needed to put on my work clothes and head in.

Upon arriving at work, there were already a few patients on the tracking board. An ambulance pulled in right behind me, and I figured that was our first burn patient.

No.

The person on the ambulance came in because her tooth hurt.

So I waited around until a second ambulance arrived.

EMS wheeled the patient in on a gurney. We couldn't tell how bad he was from the camera view, but there were several EMTs tagging along, so I didn't think the patient was in great condition.

Some men from the fire department came through the front doors.

"How many were in the house?" my coworker asked.

"Just that one," a firefighter responded.

Luckily, it turns out the person giving information on the front lawn was incorrect. According to firefighters, there were no children at the residence.

Remember that.

So, anyway, I was going to head home, but the back called and needed someone to finish registering two patients. My coworker headed to the back and I thought it'd be a pretty quick process, one that would leave me to watch the empty lobby.

Well, a man walked in with three police officers.

"Jail clearance or drug screen?" I asked.

One officer shook her head. "Neither. This is the burn patient's friend."

"I can't send visitors back right now," I explained.

"He doesn't need to go back," the officer agreed.

"He has called the patient's brother, though, and he's on the way in."

No big deal.

I sent the friend to the waiting room.

A decent amount of time passed. Emergency responders were still coming in and out of the ER. Time was of extreme importance, as the patient was about to be life lined out to a hospital with a burn unit.

The man from the waiting room approached the counter.

"They said I could see my brother."

I studied him. "The cops told me you're his friend, not his brother."

"Well, I'm his brother. I told them my brother is my best friend, so maybe they were confused."

"I can't let anyone back to see the patient unless they're family."

"That's my brother. I just told you."

The man couldn't produce identification. I was pretty sure he was lying, but there wasn't a lot I could do. So I called the back and asked the patient's nurse about the situation, explaining what the cops and man from the waiting room had told me.

"I don't care if it's grandma's sister twice removed," the nurse exclaimed. "We need someone back here to start signing off on release forms."

I buzzed the man back.

A few more minutes went by, and in walked another man.

"Someone called me about my brother. He was staying in my house and there was a fire. I would've gotten here sooner, but I had to find someone to cover the rest of my shift."

"You're his brother?" asked my coworker.

He nodded.

"Well," said my coworker, "we sent your other brother back."

"I am the *only* brother," the man corrected, rather annoyed.

"Oh," I said. "Well, he's back there."

"If this is that piece of sh—. You know what? I'm so sick of him putting his nose where it doesn't belong. I'll take care of it. Can I see my brother now?"

We buzzed the man back. He wasn't back there too long.

A few seconds after we buzzed him back, we heard raised voices. Both visitors were then escorted to the lobby by one of the lingering police officers. The men were chest to chest.

"I am his brother," the man from the waiting room argued.

"You are his client," the bio-brother retorted. "You're around as long as you think he'll slip you extra for lying when he does stupid stuff like this."

"You don't even know what you're talking about."

"Then how did my house get burned to the ground?" the brother demanded.

Boy, I wish I could insert the picture of the waiting room man that I will probably have in my mind forever. He really did have that deer caught in headlights look as he silently scrambled to come up with a reply.

"What happened was," he started. "We saw a rat. Yeah. You have rats, man. Sorry to break it to you like that, but this sucker was huge. And we tried to catch it, but it ran behind the stove. So, uh, we moved the stove, but the rat was chewing through the cord. And I said, "Man, this rat's going to ruin this dude's house, and we can't let that happen." You know, because I'm respectful of you and your place. But that rat, it kept chewing. And then there was this explosion. Before I knew it, the whole kitchen was on fire. I got all the kids out."

The patient's brother gave the other man a hard stare.

"That's not how my house was set on fire."

I guess the man from the waiting room figured that was his story and he was sticking to it.

"I'm telling you, man. A rat set your house on fire."

The two men started arguing to the point of physical altercation. Luckily, an officer saw the two and came inside to break them up.

"We located the kids," the officer said to the patient's brother. "Your brother's girlfriend said the kids have been with her since five this evening."

The brother looked to the other man. "You just told me you got the kids out of the house."

"I did! She must be whacked out of her mind. See, I rescued the kids and took them over to her house."

"Right after the rat set my house on fire, right?"

"Rat?" the cop asked. "Your brother said a meth lab exploded."

"Ya'll were making meth in my house?" blew up the brother.

"No," the man from the waiting room answered, pretending to be shocked.

"I need you to go sit down," the officer said to the man. "I need to talk to the patient's brother."

"I was going to see if he can give me a ride home," he motioned to the patient's brother.

The answer to that was "no," preceded by a whole lot of curse words.

Our patient was flown to a burn unit. The fire made the front page of our local newspaper.

The rat wasn't mentioned in the article.

A college kid came in with an X-ray request because she was trying to take selfies by tossing her camera in the air as she was lying on the bed, and I guess gravity decided to exact revenge because the camera landed on the bridge of her nose.

The girl's nose wasn't broken. She was fine.

A little stupid, but fine.

(More) Things We Want to Tell Patients/Families

** If you tell me you're our patient's brother, sister, mother, father or relative, what that means is you either came out of the same vagina or penis, the patient came out of your vagina or penis, or you're the patient's mother's/father's sister. Don't give me this, "She's my sister because we've lived in a dorm for two months" BS. That makes her your roommate, not your sister. If you're the patient's best friend and family is 11 hours away, tell us THAT, because the nurses, doctors, and even registration clerks want the patient to have someone there.

** "My mother was in the ER for an hour. We still didn't know what was going on. All the nurses were just sitting around, talking."

Ummm...all the nurses were sitting around, talking, because they didn't know what was going on, either. Test results aren't usually immediate. X-rays, CT scans, blood work...all of these things take time to come back, in addition to being passed down the chain of command. Oh, and by the way, you're not the only patient in this hospital. We want your family to be comfortable, but keep in mind we all have work to catch up on from hours before you arrived.

** "I brought my mom in because she had vaginal bleeding/breast lumps, but I had to sit in the waiting room."

Do you want to see your mom's va-jay-jay as she's put up in stirrups and given a gynecological exam? Do you want to see someone examining your mother's breasts or your father's penis to see what those 'little white bumps' are? There are times nurses use discretion as to who's allowed in the room. Yes, patients can request someone to tag along, but I doubt your mom wants you to be around when that's happening, either.

** If at all possible, leave your children with a sitter, your spouse, or someone you trust. In many cases, children under the age of 13 are not allowed in the back. Children also become bored easily, and all too often, bored children throw tantrums or are allowed to run wild, disrupting grieving or worried families.

** The other night, I received a call from a woman. She said, "I know I said my grandma was coming by car, but now she decided to go on the ambulance. I just wanted to tell you so you could tell your doctors to

47

come in out of the cold. They don't have to wait anymore."

Okay. This seems to be a common misconception around here. Maybe other hospitals have surplus staff to send out front to wait, but unless you call and say you're half a block away, nobody's going to be waiting around for patients. It's not that we don't know or don't care about a patient's condition. See, it's a simple matter of having four nurses and 20 patients, with a full waiting room. Calling ahead means nothing. We take patients as they arrive and based on the severity of the presented condition.

** Some of those hospital shows on TV aren't so far-fetched...at least in terms of the drama that takes place in a hospital. Yes, staff members form cliques. Yes, doctors are having affairs with floor nurses. Yes, people have been fired for drinking on the job. It happens. That part is reality. It happens in every industry.

** I acknowledged you before you were all the way inside. I asked how we could help you. You were registered and didn't have to wait in line before you were triaged. Your visit lasted 30 minutes. So HOW on this green and holy earth can you submit a survey that scored this hospital a negative in the time it took for staff to notice you?

** Again, this is a hospital. I know the beds seem to be mighty comfortable, the televisions have cable set up, there's free wi-fi, and you can get just about any kind of food you request, but unless you have a real emergency, you don't need to be here.

** What would possess you to ask the nurse four times if the doctor recommended that medicine? Who else do you think gave the order? I've never seen a nurse run down to the switchboard operator and ask for dosage advice.

** Are we sure that paper cut is a true medical emergency?

** Yes, I know you've been in here eight times in two days. Nope, it doesn't look busy. But it's true there will sometimes be a waiting time of at least a half hour. They like to refer to it as, 'sit there and think about why you're here.'

** "Duh."

** Unless you're bleeding to the point of passing out, are missing a limb, are having a heart attack, have someone in your party with the inability to breathe (and I don't mean 'she's short of breath,' but by the time she's at the counter, she's telling me everything that's happened to her in the last two decades), or have severe burns, wait in line like everyone else. Don't butt in front of five people and interrupt my job to tell me you want to be registered because your fingernail is numb.

** Tell your visitors to stop coming in and out so much. They either want to be with you or they don't. A periodic smoke break or stepping outside to notify family isn't really a big deal, but you don't need 800 people tag-teaming to see you because you hit your toe on the coffee table.

** "Hey, you dare me to...?" "Hey, hold my drink," and, "Hey, do you think I can...?" are all 'you're about to end up in the ER' words.

** For the love of all things holy...If you order a pizza while you're working at or just visiting the hospital, tell them your first and last name, give them your cell number, and give them a floor. We have enough to do already, and if I'm too busy, I'm not helping the pizza guy find you. (Sorry!)

** If you never ask, never say please, and never thank me for opening the doors to let you back with your family or friend, don't be surprised if I let you walk right up to those doors before I push the button and let you get smacked in the face.

What also comes along with this is: you don't own this place. I don't own this place. We have certain regulations in place that prevent even nurses or doctors from passing through certain 'shortcuts' if a patient is present. Ask if you can go back before trying to cut through.

** It's okay to request a different doctor or request a specific doctor...providing there's a choice when you come in. You don't need to tell me why. Someone may eventually ask your reasoning. You're not obligated to explain. To be honest, every nurse, registration clerk, lab tech, CNA, respiratory therapist, and ER doctor I know has a list of doctors they don't want working on them. Remember, though: if it's a true emergency, take what you can get and be thankful you have someone working so hard to keep you alive.

Get in My Belly (and Stay There)

It was a particularly rough night. Three patients coded and died in the department, including a child. On top of those deaths, we were slammed for five hours straight, and all of us were on the verge of walking out.

Let me tell you something...

When a really *special* patient registers when you're having this kind of night, it can go a few ways.

First, you can hit your limit on tolerance and being professional.

Or you can remain professional and keep your mouth shut.

I tried to do the second thing.

This young patient approached the desk and four in the morning.

"What seems to be the problem?"

"I took a pregnancy test last week. It came back positive."

I nodded.

"But ever since two days ago, I can't eat some food. I don't know why. And some foods, I used to like, but now I don't. Like, my boyfriend wanted to share his pickles with me, but I smelled them and threw up. I tried to just eat Subway, but I kept throwing it up. I need to be seen because I'm pregnant and I can't let my baby starve, and I really need Subway because I like it."

I blinked at the patient a couple hundred times.

"You're pregnant and you are having food aversions and sickness?"

She nodded.

"Yes. I need to be seen because I don't know what's wrong with me."

"And you said you're pregnant?"

She nodded again.

I wanted to repeat that she was pregnant 900 times to see if she would start to see a correlation between the baby and her symptoms, but it was obvious she didn't understand. There I was, thinking morning sickness and the inability to tolerate certain foods were common-sense symptoms of pregnancy.

Guess not.

Candid Camera

Every now and then, some of the stories that come through this ER aren't the highlight of a happy mood, but the stories that come along with them are.

My coworker and I were listening to a police chase on the scanner. The subject, I guess, was trying to flee cops by putting the pedal to the metal and going 80-something through residential areas.

This already sounds like a fantastic idea, right? I mean, when the cops tell me to stop, I'm all like, "Oh no I won't," because I highly enjoy getting tased and slammed to the ground. Oh, and I like getting arrested, too, with a huge bond and the very real possibility of going to prison.

Oh. That's not me. That was the driver.

But we're getting ahead of ourselves, aren't we?

Anyway, the driver's car was described, and the cop read the personalized license plate over the radio. It was something 'cute,' like LUVUNME99 or something that pretty much gave away that the driver was a girly girl. Now there's nothing wrong with that license plate or being a girly girl, but it sure set up the imagination to play the scene.

"It flipped. It flipped," the cop shouted.

My coworker and I groaned.

Guess which hospital was getting another patient?

The car wrecker's brother got there before she did. He seemed...antsy. Antsy, as in... maybe he was high on meth and I don't know how he even got to the ER, and he really didn't want to talk to the cops or see the cops, and he thought the security guy was a cop so he tried to run outside, but he was so high that his run was like a mixture between a penguin waddling and a turkey trying to fly. (Yes, that was meant to be a super-long sentence. Try to read it all in one breath, really fast, and then you'll understand how that woman's brother was speaking to us.)

We don't know where the patient's brother ran off to, but the ambulance arrived with the wrecker, right around the same time the cops pulled up out front.

Once the cops disappeared to the back, the patient's brother came back inside and paced the lobby.

"Heard she wrecked," he said. "She wrecked, huh?"

We almost didn't realize he was talking to us. He never made eye contact, and his words weren't loud enough to think he was doing anything but talking to himself.

"That's what I heard," I answered.

"So, uh, how's the car? Is it bad? Know where I can pick it up?"

Um, we actually get this question a lot. Let's go ahead and make this clear: you're asking a hospital registration clerk. I would think the person to ask is the towing company, the impound, or a police officer.

"I don't know," I answered.

55

"Did they, uh, check the trunk? Did they say anything about the trunk?"

Ding, ding, ding.

Those were the bells going off in my head that maybe we had a reason for running from the cops, in case you haven't guessed.

While I was preparing my paperwork to go see the car wreck patient, a woman with stringy, greasy hair and three teeth ran inside the foyer, knocked on the part of the glass doors that don't open, and motioned for the patient's brother to follow. I'm still not sure why she didn't walk the extra foot to where the doors opened, but maybe that's another story.

Before I knew it, the patient's brother was gone.

I went to the back to gather information.

Two nurses were standing outside the patient's room, speaking to the arresting officer. One nurse was inside the room. I could tell by her tone that she didn't have much patience left.

So I walked in the room.

"Tell them," she said, trying to sit up as she reached out to me, "that I shouldn't have to go to jail because it's almost my birthday."

I skipped over that and tried to ask the patient registration questions, but she wasn't having any of it.

"Where's my family?"

I explained to the patient that her brother was in the lobby, but he left.

"Nobody loves me," she blubbered.

I heard some commotion in the hall. Since I was

getting nowhere with the patient, I left the room.

Our janitor was excitedly speaking to the cop and nurses.

According to the man, he recently purchased and installed a home security system, complete with exterior cameras. He could watch and review his cameras on his phone, and when he heard the gossip of the car chase near his residence, he reviewed his tapes.

Yep, the patient's car went around the corner and flipped...right in the janitor's front yard.

In the end, the patient was carted to jail.

As soon as the cops opened the trunk, a warrant went out for the patient's brother and that girlfriend.

They were later arrested for distributing the heroin that filled up part of the patient's trunk.

Oh, oh.

I forgot, the patient's excuse for running from the cops:

"I wasn't running from the police. I just didn't see them for, like, thirteen blocks."

The cop said, "Then maybe I should get a few more of those flashing lights to put on the top of my squad car."

One of the nurses told me he was checking vitals of a woman knocked out on a morphine drip, when the nurse farted. The noise was so loud and the smell so rancid that the patient woke up, asked what the noise was, and inquired about the smell.

The nurse said he didn't know what sound the patient heard, but he didn't hear it.

And then he said the smell was coming from a potty chair in another patient's room.

32 Teeth Discount

I was down in the cafeteria after clocking out one morning, and I saw a man at the made-to-order omelet bar. He was ordering three ham and cheese omelets, with a side of hash browns.

After a 12-hour shift, all I could think about was loading up a Styrofoam takeout tray with biscuits and gravy before high-tailing it home, so I lost sight of the patient while I tried to make this happen.

I snapped my tray closed and rooted through the cooler for juice.

When I turned around, I saw the man from the omelet bar holding a Styrofoam tray with his left hand, while he used his right hand to shovel his omelets in his mouth.

Yes, it was an odd sight.

No, I've never witnessed anyone tossing omelets in his/her mouth in the center of the cafeteria.

I made it to the register before the man did, and I started to pay for my meal and drink.

Since there wasn't a line at the omelet bar, the cook left that station, crossed the cafeteria, opened a register, and called the man over to ring up.

And I kid you not, this next part really happened.

When the man approached the counter, the cashier

punched in an order of three ham and cheese omelets and hash browns.

This is when the guy flipped out.

"You can't charge me for three omelets," he screamed. "There's only one in the box."

Yes. Yes, the man ate two of the omelets before he reached the register.

And yes, the man was honestly trying to pay for one omelet. He was adamant that he not be charged for the two he consumed.

The food service manager was called in to intervene, but the man wouldn't budge with his argument. Security was then paged.

In the end, the house supervisor brushed off the charges.

That wasn't enough for the man.

He also demanded a free omelet for the 'discrimination' and 'trouble' the hospital put him through.

When the man became violent and began tossing pre-packaged sandwiches from the coolers, the police were called in.

Our food fighter was arrested for possession of methamphetamine and tested positive for the drugs as well.

<u>Untitled</u>

I don't even have a good title for this one because I'm still kind of grossed out.

So, I was trying my hardest to get out of going to the back to finish registering a few patients, but I pulled the short straw and made my way to the first patient's room.

There was really nothing interesting to see in the first three rooms.

The last room was a different story.

When I saw the patient's chief complaint was an abrasion to his forehead, I figured it'd be an in and out thing.

Upon entering the room, I prayed it would be.

Here was this man, so heavily intoxicated I was pretty sure I was getting buzzed just from him opening his mouth to speak. But that wasn't what I noticed first.

What I noticed was this man was lying on the cot with his legs spread, as if he had them in stirrups. He had a thin sheet covering his lower body, and he wasn't wearing a shirt.

I tried to get the man's information.

"I don't give that out to no one," he said, when I tried to get his real name to replace the Doe status.

I then asked if he'd give me his SSN to find him in the system.

"I don't give that out to no one, either."

"Can I get your address for correspondence?"

Want to guess his answer?

That's right. He 'don't give that out,' either.

But the patient did start asking me his own counter-questions.

He asked my name. He asked about my relationship status. He asked where I lived, what kind of car I drove, what kind of movies I like, and asked about my job.

I refused to answer his questions.

"Sir, can you give me any kind of contact information so the hospital can reach you?"

The man began lifting the sheet over his lower body.

He was completely nude.

"Like what you see?" he asked, as he flapped the sheet. "Bet you like what you see."

What I saw was something that kind of resembled a shriveled up Vienna sausage with too much extra casing at the end. It was resting atop two lopsided testicles that resembled rotten flattened peaches.

"Sir," I said with a sigh, "it's clear you don't want to cooperate, so I hope you get to feeling better."

As I started to walk out of the room, the man yelled out a phone number.

"I usually don't give that out to no one, but call me

some time," he flirted.

The patient wasn't around for too much longer. He left the hospital completely naked...and was arrested for public intox and indecent exposure.

If you're going to make a trip to the hospital's coffee shop, make sure you're not so high you try to reach through the glass cooler front to grab a soda.

I'm sure all the recently-clocked-out ER people in line with me were thrilled to have to get a bloody, whacked out man screaming because his arm hurt and he was still thirsty back to the emergency room for treatment.

Trivia Question:

Do you know why there are signs on bridges that read, "Slow down," or, "Bridge Ices Before Road," or, "Watch for Ice"?

It's because you should slow down and watch for ice that forms on the bridge before the road. Those signs aren't suggestive.

Around here, bridges are slicker than snot during winter, yet so many people heading to or from work or home seem to think nothing of it.

During winter, our ER's highest traffic happens around factory shift changes. We go from seeing maybe five patients to seeing 15 or 20, most brought in via ambulance after their vehicle has been totaled.

Trust me on this one. Slow down before your tires hit the bridge. Depending on sky conditions, a flight team may not be able to transfer you, or the flight may be delayed. The same goes for an ambulance ride to fix your 27 broken bones.

In all the time I've worked at a hospital, I've heard drunk drivers cry for several reasons.

Reasons why they cry:

The cops found out.
Their parents were going to find out.
They wrecked their car.
Their insurance is going to go up.
They don't have bail money.
They are going to lose their jobs.
They can't afford the fines.
They're going to lose their licenses.
It ruined their plans for the night.
It ruined their plans for the weekend.
They're going to lose custody of their kids.

What I've never heard a drunk driver cry about:
They could have killed someone.
They **did** kill someone.

Something I learned from working in the ER:

You apparently CAN lose your belly button ring inside of your body.

I didn't believe the patient until I heard a doctor tell a nurse to get a suture cart ready because he was going to have to cut a chunk of the patient's flesh away from her belly button in order to retrieve the ring.

She left with her belly ring in a specimen jar and with eight stitches around her navel.

Vehicle injuries are a common occurrence. Most people overlook the dangers in turning their backs to the door as they're loading up kids or groceries.

I've registered lots of patients with the complaint of being hit in the head, back, legs, ankles, and neck when the car door slammed shut because of wind or another force.

Ladies, it's also worth noting one woman came in for a SANE kit (sexual assault) because as she was loading her belongings in the car outside of the store she closed that night, a man came up and slammed the door so hard that the first hit fractured her tibia and the second blow landed against her skull, rendering her unconscious.

She's Got a Feelin'

I sometimes feel like anyone in the healthcare industry deserves a special award for memorizing the, 'don't worry, we've seen it all speech' and performing said speech at least three times a week.

When a teen patient approached the front desk, she was hobbling in a squat position, with her legs spread open. The girl was crying hysterically.

"What's going on right now?" I asked.

She rested her forehead on the registration counter and sobbed.

"I need help," she cried.

"What brings you in today? Are you hurting someplace? Have you been hurt by someone?"

She shook her head.

"No. Nobody's hurt me."

"Can you tell me what's going on?"

"No," she wept. "I just need to see a doctor right now."

I explained, "I have to have some sort of chief complaint to get you registered. Can you tell me what's going on?"

She turned red. "No. No. It's so embarrassing. I

can't tell anyone. I just need a doctor."

And I kicked that speech in gear.

"Trust me: we've seen everything you can possibly imagine. We've seen things you only think happen on TV. If you can tell me what's wrong, your complaint will give the nurses and doctors a hint at what type of room you need. We don't want to put you in the wrong type of room and have to move you when you're already uncomfortable."

I thought the girl was going to tell me what her problem was, but she cried harder.

I was so close to putting 'upset' as the chief complaint, but she blurted something out.

"I have something stuck inside of me," she whispered.

I nodded. "Vaginal or rectal?"

Snot shot out of the patient's nose and splattered all over the counter.

"You mean people actually come in for this kind of stuff?" she exclaimed. "If you ask that, that must mean other people say it, too, right?"

"Yep," I replied. "I've heard it all. The nurses and doctors in the back have seen it all. There's no need to feel embarrassed about anything. Everyone is here to help you feel better."

The girl's sobs became light sniffles.

"I, uh, have something stuck, uh..."

She looked away and then back to me. The girl leaned over the counter.

"I have something stuck in my, uh...Up my butt."

I finished registering the patient and noted she was quickly moved from the Tracking Board to a private room designed for complaints such as 'FB (foreign body) in rectum.'

The patient did the same squat waddle to the back and I didn't think much of it.

Then the phone rang.

"I'm about to go in thirteen. Did you call her mom for consent?"

I glanced over to the Tracking Board.

Crap. She was a minor.

"Sorry," I said. "I must have been distracted by the complaint."

"It's okay. I'll call her parents."

I thought that part was said and done, but then I heard the girl screaming 'no' repeatedly and begging the nurse not to call home. By law, however, the patient's parents were required to be notified.

The girl's mother worked nearby. She arrived at the hospital 10 minutes later.

Mom, of course, seemed worried. She didn't know what would lead her child to registering at the ER. Mom stated she went to work and left the patient alone, given the patient was in high school and could take care of herself.

The patient's mother asked me why her daughter was admitted to the ER, but I couldn't bring myself to tell her. Instead, I told her she could go back to the patient's room because it was best that she heard the story from her daughter.

I let the patient's mother back, but I realized I forgot to take the patient's registration paperwork to the unit clerk, so I headed back at the same time.

"Are you okay?" the mother asked the patient.

I couldn't help but to stand at the unit clerk's area and listen to the exchange. Two nurses in the patient's room had the same look on their faces as I had on mine.

"No, I'm not okay," the girl shouted. "I'm in the emergency room, mom."

"Well, what happened? You stay alone all the time. What happened?"

"I can't tell you."

"Tell me. You're here. There's no turning back now."

I craned my head forward. I saw the patient's bare abdomen jiggling.

Hmm...

"I can't, mom."

Mom was beginning to lose patience. "If you don't tell me, you're getting an automatic grounding. We can start with three weeks."

"But if I tell you, you're going to be mad."

Mom shrugged. "But if you tell me and it's not horrible, you may not be in any trouble. Just tell me what happened."

"I, uh," the patient stammered. "I was, uh, experimenting."

"You're in high school. What do you mean you

were experimenting? Did you have friends over after I explicitly told you not to? Oh my God. Are you high?"

"No. Why don't you trust me?"

"Probably because you're in the ER right now," mom retorted. "I'm getting tired of messing around. Tell me what happened."

"I used your vibrator to try anal, and—."

Mom interrupted, "You did what? Are you kidding me? Are you freaking kidding me right now?"

"I just wanted to try it," the patient yelled. She was near tears again.

"So why are you here?" mom asked. "Did you tear or something?"

The girl shook her head.

"Then what happened?"

"It got stuck. Now I can feel it right here," she said, touching her fingertips to her lower abdomen.

Mom walked to the patient's bed and placed her hand where the patient had touched.

"I can feel it," mom exclaimed. "It's still on? I can feel it."

Yeah. The vibrator was still on. It also traveled so far that it was lodged in the patient's colon, which meant it had to be removed surgically.

Surprisingly, the patient's family seemed supportive. They were also embarrassed, but I think, overall, they were happy that the patient made it through surgery okay.

Free Tip:

If you're going to be using a hand sander to smooth down a woodworking project, you should probably 1.) have your clothes on, 2.) not drink 14 beers before you start, and 3.) keep the thing away from your penis.

One man learned that the hard way.

<u>Inside the Fire</u>

Patients' families sometimes don't understand that a lot of staff members they encounter cannot lawfully comment on a patient's condition. Sure, the X-ray tech may know in her mind 200% that a patient broke a bone—either because she takes thousands of X-rays a year or there's this little bitty hint, like the bone is snapped in half and neither part touches the other—but by law, she can't tell you it's broken.

See, the same thing goes for a lot of people in the hospital. It's a liability thing.

I was counting the hours, minutes, and seconds until my shift would be over when a van pulled up in front of the ER entrance. Someone jumped out from the driver's side passenger seat and hit the emergency notification button on the exterior portion of the ER. This action, of course, sounded an alarm throughout the emergency room, and the triage nurse hurried to meet the person.

The woman who'd hit the button ran inside and screamed, "She needs help. My mom needs help right now."

"What kind of problem are we dealing with right

now?" asked the triage nurse.

"She done fell in a fire. It's bad."

Now, when people use those words ("It's bad."), I kind of want to roll my eyes because 99.99% of the time, it's really not that bad.

In this case, I could tell it was bad. As soon as the triage nurse opened the passenger door of the van, she turned right back around, ran inside, and ordered me to call the back. She needed assistance and she wanted me to tell the remaining nurses in the back to prepare a trauma room and bring out the burn cart.

Three more nurses ran outside with a stretcher after I notified the back. It took all three of them and the triage nurse to carefully transfer the patient from the van to the stretcher. Even though the doors were closed, I could hear a woman shrieking in agony.

I popped the door to allow the hurried nurses to get the patient to the back. As they passed through the lobby, I noted the patient's bare skin was charred and bleeding in most areas between her chest and knees.

The driver came inside.

"She's drunk. Her husband just died. She lives in a cabin out in the country and decided to start a campfire and sit outside and drink. But she fell in the fire."

"Wow," I replied.

"She called me four times, but I never saw the missed calls," the woman continued. "She's been unconscious in the snow, burned, for three hours. I'm a horrible daughter."

I tried to assure the woman that she wasn't a bad

daughter.

"Should I call my brothers and sisters? It's not that bad, right?"

This is when that opening statement came into play. I knew, without a doubt, the elderly patient was going to be transferred out. I also knew the patient sustained severe burns to a large portion of her body, and I knew what could accompany burns like that: shock and infection. I've heard of people dying for less serious burns.

I explained to the patient's daughter that I was unable to give her a concrete answer, but it was my personal recommendation that she should call her family. I stated it was also my personal opinion that the patient would be transferred to another hospital. The patient's daughter understood and took to making calls.

A while later, the patient's other daughters and sons arrived. I told them two could go back at a time, and I would escort the chosen two to the patient's room. When I walked two daughters to the room, one stopped me from walking away.

"Stay," she begged. "I need to use the restroom after I find out what's going on, and I'll need you to show me where it is."

I didn't have a lot going on at the time, so I didn't mind sticking around.

As I stood outside the room, I could hear the patients' daughters asking about her condition.

"I can't tell you she's not going to die," the doctor told the daughters. "Your mother has sustained burns to approximately ninety-percent of her body."

I don't know if the daughters were just in shock or if they really didn't understand.

"But I've burned myself before, and my skin always heals," one of the women argued.

The doctor hesitated. "Your mother sustained deep, third-degree burns. The flame literally burned her nerve endings in several locations. Her intoxication levels are through the roof, and that's actually helping her right now. Her body is in shock. I hate to tell you this, but I would personally consider bringing in your family and appreciating the moments you have with your mother, at least until the chopper gets here and we fly her out."

I moved and faced the room. I could see one of the daughters holding her mother's burned hand. She squeezed her hand and clear fluid seeped from the patient's burn and dripped to the floor.

The patient was intubated and a helicopter was called.

It took three other nurses and the rest of the patient's family to explain to the women why their mother may not live.

The patient lived for two more days, but her burns proved too severe for her body to handle.

We hear a lot of stories that don't make the best sense.

An example of this is the patient with a chief complaint of 'decided to take flashlight in shower with me, slipped, and now can't get the flashlight out of my butt."

Make a Run for It

We all thought we were lucky that night, because we hadn't registered a single patient since our shift began. The hours crept by. Nurses in the back were singing Three Dog Night songs at the top of their lungs and who knows where the auxiliary departments were.

To be honest, it was a great night. We were desperate for a break after a week of losing patients nearly every single shift.

Then four rolled around and an ambulance pulled in the bay.

And the patient was naked.

And screaming.

And bleeding.

And drunk.

Yay!

This man swore up and down he was 'minding his own business, trying to be a good citizen' (only he didn't say citizen, he said certification), when he was attacked by a stray cat as he was walking home from the bar. He allegedly ran from the cat, but the beast was relentless. (Yeah, he actually used that line, although it came out as one big slur.) The man came to the conclusion that the cat was attracted to the smell of his clothes, so the man continued running and stripped nude while doing so. After running for two blocks, the man was out of breath. He thought he lost the cat, but much to his surprise, the cat somehow ended up in front of the man, and it attacked again, scraping its nails down the front of the man's chest so hard and deep that the lacerations required 18 stitches.

I'm sure that's how it all happened. I mean, really, that sounds like a legitimate story, right?

Anyway, lab went in to draw the man's blood. They told him they were just going to test his BAC and make sure he didn't have elevated blood cell counts.

I'm guessing the first part of the lab tech's explanation was what scared the patient.

He ripped his IV out as soon as the first tube of blood was drawn, and he tore off his gown.

(What was it about being naked for this guy?)

The patient then drunkenly sprinted out of his room and down the ER halls. Nurses and doctors chased after him.

The patient tried to escape the ER by heading toward the exit doors.

Let me give you a quick rundown of how these doors work. See, they're pretty simple to operate. You press a button located on the wall, and then the doors open automatically. If you don't press the button, you *can* open them, but I've seen 300-pound-men struggle with the feat.

And let's go back to our 140-something-pound

patient, who was showing no signs of slowing down as he ran toward the double doors.

No, he didn't hit the button.

No, he didn't extend his arms to push through the doors.

This man was under the impression that the doors swung open easily, and he could run right through them.

Ha ha...

Yep, you got it. The patient hit those doors face first and ricocheted backward. He fell flat on his bare bottom.

The patient ended up breaking three teeth and his nose in the bolt.

When the doctor asked the man why he ran, the patient responded that he was 'really drunk' and thought he was going to jail.

We explained to the man that because he wasn't picked up by the cops and he wasn't wanted for committing a crime, he wasn't in danger of being arrested.

His BAC came back about three times the legal limit. He was released to his sister.

Cold as Ice

Lately, several states have declared disaster areas due to flooding. In our area, bridges were shut down due to log jams, empty fields flooded and took out miles upon miles of roads, and all of this meant what once took what seemed like forever to get to the nearest city in the first place was extended by the need to take detours around all the flooding.

And then, if you were paying attention to the news, you may have noticed that shortly after weeks of rain, winter decided to knock the 60s out of the way and come in with teen temperatures and lots of snow.

These things don't mix well.

We were all huddled around the police scanner one night, listening to a police chase.

According to officers, someone noticed a gas station employee in the town over started her car to thaw out the windows. The man saw an opportunity and took it. Then he was on the run, well, as much of a run as he could manage on icy country roads, anyway.

It was a steady chase, I think. The officer in pursuit couldn't go any faster, and neither could the thief. Another officer called over an order to simply follow the car thief and apprehend the criminal once the car stopped or wrecked.

Easy enough, right?

Things took a turn for the worse.

"The vehicle is spinning out of control on [a well-known bridge separating two counties]," the officer announced.

"Oh! Oh! I need help now. I need help. The vehicle has gone over the bridge. I repeat, I need help. The vehicle has gone over the bridge and is now in the river. I'm going to move in on foot and see what I can do."

Dispatch started calling in EMTs and firefighters.

"I can't see the car," the officer panicked, nearly out of breath. "But there's someone in the water. He's screaming that the driver is still in the car."

The scanner was hopping with conversation.

"I can't get this guy out of water. I can't."

A nearby farmer, I guess, saw and heard the commotion from his home and drove his tractor to the river bed. He then thought quickly and tossed a rope to the weakened, injured criminal. The farmer dragged the man out of the water, over a sheet of ice, and stayed with him after the man collapsed on the shore.

EMS came over the radio a few minutes later and announced the man would be transported to our hospital. He was in shock, was unconscious, and he sustained obvious trauma to his head, neck, back, legs, and arms...and that was just what EMS could see.

When the patient arrived at the hospital, he was

warmed up slowly and was flown out due to a broken collarbone, two broken legs, cracked ribs, and doctors were concerned because the patient had water in his lungs.

The man did live and is awaiting sentencing for his role in the car theft.

His friend, on the other hand, became trapped in the car and drowned. It took a crew from an inner city to retrieve the stolen car from the river.

Polish the Pole

Sometimes a type of injury on one patient will seem hilarious, while the same type of injury on another patient seems horribly unfair.

For example, a young boy, not even in double digits yet, was brought in by EMS for a rectal/buttock injury. While running through the backyard, chasing after the family dog, the boy stepped on the metal portion of a garden tool lying on the ground and somehow fell. The tool's wooden handle impaled the child rectally. This patient lived, but it was difficult to see such a young boy in so much distress. And, of course, we were all concerned for the child's future, as his rectum was left tattered, essentially, from the accident.

To all of us, the accident was senseless and tragic.

When an adult male came in with a similar...complaint...it was a little more difficult for some of us to keep a straight face when we were out of the room. Sure, we felt bad for the man, but the back story kind of set the scene that night.

This middle-age man was brought in via ambulance. He was positioned face-down on a stretcher, and EMS tried to give the man what dignity they could by draping a sheet over his buttocks. Well, because there was something protruding from his buttocks, part of the sheet rested on the man's back, then the center part of the sheet was about as high in the air as the length of my arm, and the other part of the sheet rested against the man's thighs.

The man was crying, yet trying to breathe evenly and stay calm like EMS kept telling him.

"What happened here?" asked a nurse, just back from her break.

"He, uh, says he fell," one of the EMTs answered. "He fell on the leg from a dining room chair and now can't get the leg out. We had to cut it from the chair to transport him."

The nurse started to get wide eyes, but the patient looked up to see her reaction and she quickly just bit her lip and nodded.

This man was moved to a trauma room, where the real story came out.

It's not difficult to imagine what happened here, but I'll spell it out in case some of you have pure minds.

He decided to pleasure himself by turning a dining room chair upside down and sitting on one of the legs. He stated he lost his footing and fell, pushing the chair leg up much further than he expected.

It wasn't easy for the nurses and doctors to assess the situation. When they finally did, they had to explain to the patient that he would have to go to surgery as soon as possible. His bowel was perforated, and the force of the fall caused internal bleeding.

Then the man requested that someone call his wife.

87

She was out of town that weekend, staying with her sister for a bachelorette party.

The couple is still together. The patient's recovery took some time, but he seems to be doing well, although he's still using a colostomy bag and says he may have to wear it the rest of his life.

Is your hospital so dry that you're getting shocked endlessly throughout the winter months?

I swear, the other day I hit the button to open the doors and am pretty sure I was partially electrocuted.

Viral Videos

It's a stretch, sure, but let's go from talking about being physically shocked to feeling emotionally shocked. (Hey, I'm trying to make it work.)

Anyway, welcome to the age of technology. Welcome to a time when it seems the majority of the population owns a mobile phone with internet capability. Welcome to the age of witnessing an accident and seeing a crowd holding up phones, recording the aftermath, rather than helping. Welcome to ordinary people doing extraordinarily dumb things to get 15 minutes of fame on YouTube or one of those television shows that shows viral video clips.

Welcome to the day and age that people will do just about anything to be famous, including trying to replicate the viral videos they've seen online or on TV.

Why people mimic these acts, I don't know. Maybe it's caused by boredom. Maybe it's caused by stupidity. Maybe it's caused by being young or carefree or just having a general curiosity of the act. But it is a problem, at least around here.

While mom and dad were away for a nice, relaxing

trip over the weekend, mom's brother was staying at the house and was responsible for watching four boys, ranging from 7 to 15.

Throughout the weekend, we learned they watched a few of the Star Wars movies, played some video games, and watched a show on cable which main premises involves showing clips of viral videos. One of those videos showcased a fairly popular 'challenge.'

If you haven't heard of the 'cinnamon challenge,' here's a quick breakdown: basically, you pour a heaping amount of cinnamon powder onto a spoon and try to swallow the powder. **Do not try this at home. Do not try this at all.** Don't get even the slightest thought in your mind that you might be able to pull it off.

In the videos, if you haven't seen them, partakers of this 'challenge' always end up in coughing fits.

But the videos don't show the depths of the dangers involved in participating.

Maybe that's why the uncle didn't see a problem when the boys challenged each other to their own 'cinnamon challenge' the night before mom and dad were due home.

So, four children and an adult lined up at the kitchen island, each with a spoon in their hands. The uncle distributed the cinnamon powder—and then some, citing 'surely' they could manage the 'challenge' – and started the countdown.

"Three, two, one..."

They were off.

All five inserted the spoons in their mouths and

tried to swallow the cinnamon powder.

The only one out of the group able to breathe clearly directly after the act was a 12-year-old. He dialed 911 before his throat closed.

Hearing five patients were coming in rattled registration. Adding five patients to an already-overloaded and short-staffed ER staff brought two nurse interns to tears.

When the patients arrived, everyone rushed to assess the acuity of each. The 12-year-old's airway was cleared by EMS and he was stable. His 15-year-old brother was hooked up to oxygen. Two stable, three to go.

The boys' uncle wasn't in great shape. He was gasping for air, and each time he coughed, flecks of cinnamon poofed into the air.

The 9-year-old of the family vomited persistently and complained of chest pain.

And then there was the youngest, a beautiful little boy with big, bright eyes and rosy cheeks. He looked like a doll, lying in his cot.

Nurses scrambled to revive the child.

Respiratory was stat paged.

One of the doctors used the defibrillator twice on the child.

Everyone prayed or crossed their fingers or hoped really hard that the child would survive.

And then he came to, vomited, and passed out again.

The boy's nurses knew he was in critical condition,

but it wasn't until other departments came in that we learned the severity of his injuries.

While waiting for EMS to arrive, the boy had a seizure, choked on even more of the cinnamon, and aspirated. The cinnamon entered his lungs and the damage was done. Both collapsed.

Our hospital rushed to arrange a helicopter for the child to be transferred to a pediatric hospital, but he was pronounced dead before the helicopter made it for transport.

We couldn't really judge the uncle because he didn't know the dangers involved in the video he watched. He saw people doing something that looked silly, and that was it. Unfortunately, one of the four children died and another was in the hospital for three months, fighting for a life he lives without handicap today because he had a great staff of dedicated nurses and doctors.

Tragedy didn't end there for the family, though.

Distraught and consumed by guilt, mom's brother committed suicide a few months later.

Man got mad because he tripped over his wife's exercise ball and spilled scalding coffee on his lap.

Man grabbed a golf club and tried to pop the exercise ball by beating it to death.

Man was knocked out cold when the golf club bounced off the ball and hit him in the head.

Exercise ball: 2.

Man: 0.

Several nurses, techs, and registration staff walked by an EMS student there to shadow. None of us knew what he was doing, so we kind of just walked away and pretended not to notice.

Finally, a doctor approached the teen, tore an ordinary desktop stapler from the guy's hands, and yelled, "What the hell do you think you're doing in my ER?"

The doctor looked down to the 19 (NINETEEN!) staples the intern shot into his own arm.

"Tell me what you were thinking," the doctor demanded.

The teen shrugged. "I just thought it would be good practice for everyone since it's kind of slow right now."

He was sent home after the staples were removed.

We never saw him again.

Timber

It's an extremely rare occasion when an injury presents with a video to show how it happened. But dang, is it a great moment when you hear there's footage!

A college kid and his friend checked in during one of my just-as-rare evening shifts. The friend was laughing hysterically, while the patient was holding a bloodied rag over his nose.

"Okay," I asked, "what happened?"

The injured young man started to speak, but his friend cut him off.

"I'll do better than telling you. I'll show you. This is the funniest crap you're going to see in your whole life."

That's a pretty loaded statement. I hoped it was true.

The patient's friend whipped out his cell phone and tapped at the screen.

"Here," he said, holding the phone up for us to see. "Watch this."

The video was a little shaky, but we could still see what was going on. Our patient was sitting at one of those U-shaped desks that stretch from one side of a college classroom to the other. I guess his friend was a few seats down, recording the patient, who was sleeping with his forehead propped up with a fist.

Then the patient started bobbing his head. In the video, we could all hear the friend snickering.

"Watch this," he whispered to someone off camera.

Before I knew it, the friend tossed a pencil at the patient. It hit him in the temple, but it didn't cause him to wake up.

More snickers.

The video went on about another 30 seconds. As time passed, the patient's head bobbed more and more, as his elbow wobbled on the desk.

"Timber," his friend called in another whisper.

And then the patient's arm gave out, causing his face to crash against the desk.

Boy, that sure woke him up.

Our patient's screams were caught on film, but they were barely audible amongst the startled screams of unsuspecting students and the laughter of those around him.

The patient broke his nose in the nap accident.

Firsthand Account

For being such a small town, I'm starting to realize a lot of crazy things happen around here. I guess I never really thought much of all of these occurrences until I started recalling them in print, but as I go through years of memories, I now see that I've seen and heard some fairly wild things. Life in the ER, right?

Now, nurses and doctors may experience this more than registration clerks...I mean, it's not too often someone's on the way to work, witnesses a bad accident, and beats the ambulance to work before dealing with the patient a while later. But that's exactly what happened to my coworker.

Every now and then, every last one of the hospital workers have been caught up by one of the eight million trains that run through the center of town every day. So when my coworker was late, I figured that's where she was.

She came in about 20 minutes after her scheduled clock in time, and she was shaking from head to toe.

"What's wrong?"

She struggled to steady her breathing.

"I just saw an accident," she said. "It was bad, I

think. It had to be bad. I don't think they could've lived through it."

Well, that's a pretty good way to catch someone's attention.

"Where did it happen?"

My coworker had to sit down to tell the story because her nerves were so frazzled.

According to her, she was the first car stopped at the train tracks when the arms came down and the red lights started flashing. She noticed a truck on the other side of the tracks only slowed momentarily.

She was already crying.

"I don't know what this guy was thinking," she blubbered. "I saw him. I saw him. He looked down the tracks and saw the same train I did. He had to have known he didn't have enough time."

My coworker continued her story after a few minutes of hard sobbing.

"He pulled around the arm and tried to make it."

Tried.

The train plowed into the driver's side of the pickup and dragged it 50 feet down the tracks. Knowing she couldn't help the patient, she dialed 911 on her cell phone and, in a panic, told the operator she was late to work and would give a statement to officers later. She then put her car in reverse, drove down a few blocks, and came to work a different route.

We received two patients from that wreck. Both lived and had nothing wrong with them except a few bumps and bruises, mostly to their facial regions from the airbags deploying. Luckily for the husband and wife, the train hit directly behind the driver's seat. Neither knew why they were still alive or how they made it through such a traumatic event.

My coworker met with the patients and was overjoyed that they made it through the accident in good health.

The husband swore he'd never try making that move again.

Last Halloween, we were told registration clerks could wear costumes.

My boss, knowing my sense of humor quite well, looked directly at me and said, "No grim reaper, and no Doctor Kevorkian."

Damn.

Some Bonfire Tips

1.) If you plan to start a bonfire, make sure you can keep the fire contained. It helps if you keep the fire area bordered by stones, but if you can't, you should definitely keep it away from wooded areas and dry, overgrown fields.

2.) Let's go on ahead and keep our BAC below .568 if we're going to be playing with matches.

3.) Gasoline isn't the best accelerant choice.

4.) When you go up in flames, scream out. Don't breathe in.

5.) Don't try to hide your injuries by soaking in an ice bath for two hours while the field and woods outside of your house burn out of control.

I didn't see this patient, but I heard all about how the fire department had to call in two other counties to extinguish the fire that eventually burned his home to the ground. And I did hear all about how the patient's jeans melted and fused to his legs. I did hear how his nurse was directed to peel the charred denim from his body, and how patches of skin came off with it.

In addition to the hospital bills for the many reconstructive surgeries, infection control, and all the other medical necessities, the patient was taken to court by the city because it turns out his bonfire was lit during a no-burn order.

No matter how embarrassed or scared you are, ALWAYS tell your nurses and doctors the TRUTH! Yeah, taking your friend's mom's medication was a dumb idea, but if you lie to the people trying to help you, they're not going to be able to do it as well as if you just tell them what happened.

Everyone at a hospital has always seen or heard something equal to or worse than what you're hiding.

A Bunch of Tiny Pricks

An older man, living just a few blocks from the college, was sick and tired of college kids cutting through his back yard and trampling the flower garden his deceased wife worked endlessly at when she was still alive. It was all the man had, really, since the couple had no children or pets. He dedicated the rest of his life to maintaining the garden, so it was a slap in the face to catch a bunch of heathens purposely stomping on his wife's lilacs.

The man couldn't afford to erect a fence, so he went to a nearby nursery and special ordered cacti to plant around the flowers. He was proud of this idea. Surely, these plants would keep the kids out of the flowers, and if the nighttime heathens were drunk and tried to destroy the garden, they would be met by prickly pain they'd least expect in the middle of an Ohio yard.

For a few days, the cacti worked. The man noticed his wife's flowers were finally healing.

But one night, the man was woken from a dead sleep at the sound of hooting and hollering. The noise was coming from his back yard.

The elderly man ran outside in his boxer shorts and a white tee. He said a group of college kids were hanging out in his yard, drinking beer.

Upset, the man grabbed a garden hose and sprayed the kids. When they ran, he chased after them. Sometime during the chase, he slipped on a beer can, lost his footing on the wet lawn, and landed on the row of cacti bordering the flower garden.

When the man tried to get up, he was unable to do so. His body strength just wasn't the same it used to be. So in an attempt to stand up, the man somehow flipped himself onto his stomach...and got pricked by the cacti on the front of his body, too.

A neighbor heard the commotion and dialed 911. The man was brought in via ambulance and was given a heavy dose of pain medication.

It took more than five hours to remove the cacti needles from the man's skin, and then he was admitted to the floor for observation, due to the skin agitation the needles caused.

When the man explained how the accident happened, someone from the hospital started a fundraiser to buy the man a privacy fence. Enough money was raised to install the fence, add a few flowers and a stone memorial cross to his wife's garden, and remove the cacti so the incident wouldn't occur again.

A (Made Up) Family Affair

Around the holidays, an older woman rushed to the counter and was talking a mile a minute.

"My granddaughter. They just brought her in on the ambulance. I need to go back now."

I glanced to the security monitors and told the woman, "It doesn't look like she's here yet, so if you want to have a seat—."

"They have to be here," the lady screamed. "You're a liar and you're keeping me from my family."

Then the woman went on a long tirade about how she was going to sue the hospital and I wasn't going to have a job. Security came out and tried to calm the woman. She just wouldn't listen when we repeatedly told her the ambulance hadn't arrived, even after we invited her to check out the monitors with her own eyes. She saw the same dark and empty bay we saw, but she was convinced we were lying.

The woman made several botched attempts to run to the back, but each time was thwarted by staff. Ten minutes later, she finally went to the waiting room, where she told anyone who'd listen (or was around) how we were horrible people, keeping her away from her family.

When an ambulance rolled in, we kept it hush-hush.

It was still going to be a few minutes before the woman could go back anyway, and when we saw the chief complaint for the 9-year-old girl, 'severing of wrist,' we knew those few minutes were going to be upped a bit. We didn't want to risk ticking the woman off even more.

Someone called me from the back and told me to come get the registration information from the patient's mother. I guess the situation was a serious one. The doctor on duty took one quick look at the patient and made the decision within five minutes to transfer the child to another hospital specializing in pediatric surgery and aftercare.

I told security what was going on, and they said they'd keep an eye on grandma.

I went to the patient's room, and the sight wasn't a good one. Nurses held the patient's dangling wrist as they attempted to wrap the wound to prevent contaminants from entering. She had tendons and ligaments exposed, and several of them had been tore apart.

"What happened here?" I asked the crying mother.

"She was playing with her sister," she said. "I was in the other room. God, I should've been there. They were playing ball inside and her hand went through the window when she was trying to catch it."

The mom took a breath and said, "And then, we have these strange windows. We have a thin piece of glass, but then there's another thick piece that slides up in between the two. It fell on her wrist. Oh my God. She's going to lose her hand."

Mom's panicking caused the girl to panic. "They're going to cut my hand off? Mom, you told me they could fix me."

Nurses tried to calm the patient.

"Would you like me to send grandma back for you guys?" I asked mom.

The mother raised her brows. "What?"

"Grandma," I repeated.

This caused commotion in the patient as well. "Grandma came back from heaven?"

Oh no. Oh no. Oh no.

That's all that was running through my mind at the time. I didn't know what to do or say or think.

"Her grandparents are all...uh, in heaven. She doesn't have any living grandparents."

We heard the woman from the front let out a banshee cry and the mom put her fingers to her temples.

"I can't deal with this right now. I just can't."

"That woman," she continued, "is some crazy woman from down the street. She saw my daughter walking to school one day, and we have a restraining order against her because she's convinced my kid is her grandkid. She went to school one day and told them my daughter had a death in the family, and then she tried taking her out of state to go to her family's place for a funeral that wasn't even real. The police found them at a gas station."

One of the nurses whipped her head around, "What?"

"That woman," mom said, "cannot see my daughter. I don't even know how she knows we're here, unless she saw the ambulance. I can't do this. I can't deal with this right now."

I informed security about the situation and the police were called due to the nature of the complaint.

When the police arrived, they tried to peacefully inform the older woman that she couldn't be at the hospital to visit the child, and she could have no contact with the child.

We knew there was something mentally wrong with the woman, so it was hard to judge her, especially because of her age.

In the end, the police took the woman in custody and her family flew in from Oregon or some state out west. We never saw the woman again.

The injured child went through a series of surgeries to reconnect her wrist to her arm.

If you're going to walk around the house, holding something in your mouth, try not to be clumsy and hit the wall as you're turning off the light.

A patient spent a few thousand dollars and a few hours in surgery because the kebab skewer he was holding between his lips was shoved to the back of his throat, where it penetrated his esophagus.

Ouch.

Play Ball

A man was brought to the ER via ambulance for a leg injury. According to EMS, the patient was a pain in the butt, and so much so that they basically dropped the man off, said "good luck," and hightailed it out of there.

The EMTs were so right. He was rude, crude, and inappropriate with all the nurses, asking for dirty pictures, requesting that the techs help him urinate by stroking his penis, and he threw a pillow at the X-ray tech. Wondering if the man also sustained head injuries to possibly explain his excessively poor behavior, the doctor on duty ordered a CT. There was nothing physically wrong with the man's head. He was just a jerk.

I went in the room to gather the man's information. He was a new patient to the hospital, so I knew it was going to take some time. And because I heard about his behavior, I figured it was going to take a while. He showed me his penis twice and tried to grope my breasts as I held the clipboard steady for him to sign the consent form.

"Don't touch me," I told the patient, as he tickled my arm with his free hand. "I don't like that."

The man scoffed and called me just about every

name in the book.'

I hadn't even touched down on the information yet.

Oh, it was going to be a long night.

It took 15 minutes just to drag the address, phone number, and next of kin out of the man.

"And how did you hurt yourself?" I asked.

"Baseball bat."

"Oh. Were you assaulted? Nobody said anything about that."

"Did I say I was assaulted?"

The man's knee was hanging low and to the left.

"So you hit yourself with a baseball bat?"

"Did I say that?"

I sighed.

"Sir, if you don't want to answer the questions, I'll gladly mark down that you refuse to cooperate. That will prevent me from placing your insurance on your account, if you have any, and you will receive no complimentary discount from the hospital."

"Want to catch a movie after I'm out of here?" he asked with a sly smile.

I shook my head. "No. I just want to know how you hurt yourself."

"I don't know that I want to tell anyone that."

I blew out a mouthful of hot air. "Okay. Look, if you decide you want to cooperate, let your nurse know and she'll call me. Get to feeling better."

"I was mad," the man said, as I started to walk out of the room. "I went to blow off some steam with my buddies by playing box ball."

"Box ball?" I asked, turning around.

He nodded. "It's when one person drives and there's someone in the bed of a truck with a ball bat. Whoever destroys the most mailboxes in the time frame wins and the loser has to buy us all drinks."

I bit my lower lip. "Okay."

"This one mailbox, I've destroyed it, like, fifteen times this year, right? But today, I went to knock it out of the park, and when the bat hit the box, it bounced back and hit my knee. Do you think it's broken?"

"I don't know," I responded. "But aren't you a little old to be damaging others' property?"

He shrugged. "No. But I might have to take it easy for a while, and I guess I won't try taking that box down again."

The man continued to explain the box's owner was probably tired of putting the box back time after time, so I guess he or she filled the box with cement.

The man stopped being so obnoxious for a while, but he was right back to it when he learned he was going to jail for damage to private property.

He went to jail with a patella fracture.

Had a patient come in via ambulance tonight.

Everyone rolled their eyes.

The patient lives next door to the hospital, within 100 feet of the entrance.

She called 911 for dental pain.

When she was discharged, she requested an ambulance for transport.

It took an hour for the ambulance to come, load her up, and take her back home—just a one-minute walk away.

I once registered this man who presented with a pretty bad head injury that he sustained when he tried to push on the glass gas station door.

They were in the middle of renovating, so there was no glass in the door.

The patient fell through the frame, hit his head on the floor, and he had to get 11 staples.

How to get reported by a patient and end up in a meeting with your boss:

I went outside to start my car, and as I was very carefully walking back to the entrance, hoping not slip on ice, I saw one of the ER nurses running through the parking lot, eager to get out of the freezing weather.

"I'd pay a lot of money to see you fall and bust your [butt]," I hollered to my coworker with a laugh.

And that's when a man dressed in scrubs and the same color beanie as my coworker turned around and angrily said, "What did you just say to me?"

It turned out the man worked at a local nursing home and was at the hospital because his mom was just moved to inpatient hospice.

He didn't care that I was joking, and I was mortified. My boss didn't care, either. I was in a little bit of trouble for that one.

If you're going to store sparklers in your back pocket to use on New Year's Eve, make sure your idiot friend doesn't think it'd be funny to light them while they're still in your pocket.

The college-aged victim suffered third degree burns on his buttock, as well as all the way up his back after the sparklers ignited his t-shirt.

<u>Going Downhill</u>

Last week, I saw an injury that took me back to my childhood, when my brother did something similar (and ended up with a silver-dollar-sized hole straight through his hand).

EMS brought in a screaming pre-teen. We didn't know too much about the kid's injuries or how he sustained them, but it was clear he was in pain and we were worried that it was pretty serious because dad came to the registration desk and was crying.

Dad answered all the registration questions and signed consent, but he didn't have the family's new insurance cards; mom did, but she was in the room with their son. We had to go through the accident screen, and dad let out every detail.

The family lives out in the country, I guess, and the boy was riding his bike down a gravel-coated hill with his two sisters following behind him and three of the family's dogs running ahead of the group.

Dad wasn't exactly sure what happened, but he was told by one of his daughters that the puppy of the group saw something in the small patch of woods off to the side, stopped to look, and her brother plowed right into the dog.

That wasn't all.

When the boy's bike hit the puppy, he was thrown over his handlebars, which he tried a little too hard to cling to. One of his shoulders dislocated.

Even that sounds easy enough to handle, but dad was highly upset, so we knew there was more.

The child had to land eventually. He landed on his side, head first. The child's ear was torn nearly all the way off, held to his head by less than an inch of flesh. From his chin to his temple...degloved. Three of the boy's teeth were knocked out, and one pierced through his cheek. In addition to the facial injuries, the impact of the fall to the child's chest caused a cardiac arrhythmia.

Part of working in this field, something that most people just don't seem to understand, is often not knowing what happens to these patients when they leave our facility. In some cases, it's not too difficult to ask another hospital how the patient fared—if anyone can find the time to remember to make the call or the person on the other end of that line has access to those records. The truth is, it's just one of the hard parts of a job in healthcare, worrying about a patient long after he or she has been discharged from the hospital.

In this case, a doctor called to check up on the boy. Surprisingly, he was emotionally upbeat, but physically, he was looking at multiple surgeries.

Math problem:

"I dare you to" + copious amounts of alcohol + a trampoline x (midnight and dark) + can't do what they dared you to do even when you're sober.

Solve.

Answer:

Paralysis. The female patient tried to do a back flip, fell off the trampoline, and suffered a C5/C6 vertebrae injury.

__But I Came by Ambulance!__

Even before I walked in, I knew it was going to be a busy night. There were four cop cars in front of the ER, and the waiting room was full.

When I made it inside, EMS was wheeling one of our frequent flyers out of the back and to the registration desk. His girlfriend was holding two Big Gulps and a bag of Doritos.

"This is his information," said the EMT, handing the sheet to my coworker, as if we didn't already know the man's name, birthday, address, and phone number by heart. "Have fun."

The EMT left and I was putting my stuff away.

"But I came by ambulance!" the patient yelled. "This isn't fair. You call an ambulance because you want to go straight back."

I could have kept my mouth shut, but I didn't.

"That's not how it works," I said. "If an ambulance comes in when we're busy—like we are now—and you're not facing a life or death illness, you'll be triaged like you walked through the door."

The man's girlfriend rolled her eyes. "But I called them and told them he had chest pain. We know what to say to get to the back."

"Did you tell the ambulance guys that?"

The patient nodded. "Yes."

I shrugged. "Then maybe that's why they put you out here. We have people calling 911 over all kinds of things, just to get in the back. Dental pain. Leg pain. Fever."

The patient looked confused. "Are you just naming all the reasons I was in here this month?"

I acted surprised. "Oh! That was you on those ambulances? I forgot."

"I wanted to get in and out," the man replied. "There's no crime in that."

I shrugged and walked away.

"Sir," said my coworker, "there's one patient in front of you, and then someone will take you back."

The patient said he couldn't wheel himself to the waiting room (and I don't know why, because we've seen him do it a million times before), and the patient's girlfriend showed my coworker that her hands were too full from the drinks and bag of chips. My coworker pushed the patient over to the waiting room and came back to the desk.

And the minutes passed.

Six...yes, six...minutes later, while the patient before the chest pain man was in triage and almost finished with the process, the man and his girlfriend announced they were leaving.

The triage nurse heard this.

"You're leaving? There's one person in front of you. I'm taking them back now, and then it's your turn."

"I've already waited long enough," the patient said. He was standing now. It's amazing, the miracles that occur when patients don't get their way. "I'm not sitting in that waiting room all night."

The nurse looked at the Tracking Board. "It's been six minutes, sir. You're next."

"I'm not waiting."

"So you called an ambulance to bring you here, and now you're just going to go home?"

The patient nodded. "Exactly."

The triage nurse thought this over. "So later, when you're feeling bad again, are you going to call the ambulance to bring you in?"

"Well, yeah, if I call and you're not busy," replied the patient.

Sadly, this exchange wasn't the first of its kind with this patient, and it won't be the last. It's also not exclusive to this patient. We see this a lot.

All You Can Be

I don't know what it is about the end of a shift that causes everyone in the world to flock to the ER, but it happens just about every morning, starting around 6:40. That's when the universe decides to throw the overnight shift one or two need-to-intervene-now cases, along with six or so other patients who all come in and want to be seen immediately because, 'you guys can't be that busy.'

That's what was going on when I was praying it wouldn't. There were just 20 minutes left of my long, long shift, and I was ready ta gooooo.

When a man frantically jogged through the entrance, I knew I wasn't getting lucky and getting out of there on time.

"What's going on right now?" I asked.

He was out of breath. "My mom. My mom has Alzheimer's. She must have left the house sometime last night. By the time we realized, it was too late. We found her in a field, three miles away from our house."

It was 19-degrees outside and two inches of snow had fallen throughout the night.

"She's so cold. She's blue. I don't know what to do.

What do I do? What do I do?"

I picked up the phone and dialed the charge nurse.

"We need help out here," I said. "And bring blankets."

The man ran back out to his car. His wife got out of the passenger seat and opened up the back passenger door. I could see a pair of bare feet, but the person in the back wasn't moving.

Four nurses headed outside, and the last of the four took a wheelchair.

As soon as the four were outside, it was obvious to them that the wheelchair wasn't an option. Two nurses ran back inside and went straight to the back.

A few seconds later, three ER nurses—the first two and now the charge nurse—rolled a bed outside, with the house supervisor leading the way.

The nurses worked together to get the patient out of the car and onto the bed.

"Get ICU on the phone right now," the house supervisor yelled to me as they were all passing through the double doors to the back. "Tell them we need the Bair hugger *now.*"

(I didn't know what that was at the time, but it turns out it's a heater-like accessory used to treat hypothermic patients.)

When I called ICU, I somehow managed to get the rudest, newest nurse on the floor. This is probably a-whole-nother topic, but I've noticed several of the just-out-of-school nurses are cocky and hateful. They've earned those letters under their names and make sure to let everyone know it, including the nurses who've been around for decades. Trust me, I have nothing but admiration for nurses, but I think we all can think of someone just like the nurse on the line.

"Hey, this is Kerry in ER registration."

"And?"

"We have a situation down here and need the Bair hugger as soon as possible."

Silence.

"Hello?" I asked.

"I'm here," she snapped. "I'm just trying to figure out what you want me to do about it."

"Um, maybe bring it down here? [Unique name for our house super] told me to call you guys."

"I don't have time to do something that they could send someone like you to do. I didn't go to college to take orders from a secretary."

"Can you maybe give me to someone who will? I can't leave the desk and everyone's in that room."

I was trying my very best to stay calm.

Two more cars pulled up outside the lobby and I saw our next patient hobbling inside.

"Um, nobody else has time, either, registration."

"We have a patient down here—," I said.

She hung up on me.

I won't use the words in this story that I used as it was happening.

A woman from the first of the two new cars pushed by the hobbling man and ran to the desk.

"I need help. My daughter has a fever. It was 101 when I checked it."

"Ma'am," I said, "if you want to bring her inside and have a seat on the bench next to the door, I can help you in just a minute. I have a—."

She shook her head. "Didn't you hear me? I said it was 101."

"Ma'am, we have a life or death situation in the back, and—."

"How do you know my daughter isn't dying?"

"Ma'am, just bring her—."

"Why aren't you telling someone we're here?" she screamed. "Are you stupid?"

The man behind her was clearly irritated that the mom pushed him out of the way for a fever. He shook his head as the woman continued to berate me.

And then I lost my cool for a whole 15 seconds.

"Go park your car, bring your kid inside, sit on the bench, and wait. Someone is dying right now because you won't let me finish a sentence."

The woman tried to argue with me, but I walked away and hurried to the back.

Every nurse available was in a trauma room, placing blankets over the elderly woman.

The nursing supervisor saw me standing outside the room.

"Did they bring the hugger?"

"There's a—."

"Yes or no?"

"No. This—."

"Did you call them?"

I was dangerously close to losing my temper and my job at that point.

"Yes, but—."

"So why don't we have it yet?"

"If everyone would stop interrupting me for two seconds, I could tell you the nurse up there said she doesn't take orders from a registration person, and she doesn't have time to bring it down. Then she hung up on me."

The nursing supervisor turned around and kicked over an equipment tray. Tools flew all over the place and the tray rattled as it jiggled on the tile floor. All the nurses and two doctors jumped.

The super took a deep breath and turned to me.

"I'm sorry for yelling at you. It's not your fault. We just really need that equipment."

I nodded.

"We're locking down," she told me. "Register people if they come in, but send them to the waiting room. I don't care if anyone gets mad. Nobody comes back unless they're having chest pain or they're bleeding to death, okay?"

"Okay."

"When her family comes inside, take them to the consult room or the chapel. It's not looking good."

The nursing supervisor left the room, clearly on a mission. She was running full speed out of the ER and toward the back part of the hospital, where the ICU elevators were.

I went back to the front. The furious mother was right there at the desk, holding a four-year-old.

"Do you think you took long enough?" she snapped.

I registered the child but didn't say anything to the mother about the wait until it was time to tell her to go to the waiting room.

"But it's empty," she said, waving to the room. I could see the family for the other patient smoking and hugging in the parking lot.

"I told you, we have a life or death situation in the back. I'm sorry, but all of our nurses are trying to save a patient."

"This is unbelievable," the woman growled. "Unbelievable."

She muttered the entire walk to the waiting room.

The other patients weren't as pushy. They seemed to understand the severity of the situation, but they were still irritated. One man complained that he was going to be late for work.

"I just said—." I heard, coming from down the hall.

I turned my head and saw the house supervisor carrying the hugger and walking in front of an ICU nurse.

"And I just said I don't care."

She pointed at me. "Open that door for me now and then come to the back."

I did as I was told. Honestly, and I'm not sure why, I was scared I was in trouble. Years have gone by, but never before or since have I seen that woman so angry.

She handed off the hugger to the doctors in the room and pointed to the room.

"Look at that patient," she seethed to the ICU nurse.

The nurse glanced at the woman and away again.

"Look at her," the nursing supervisor ordered. "Take a long, hard look at this woman. She has a family. She has a life. And you don't get to decide whether she lives or dies because you're too high and mighty to perform a simple task."

I could tell the ICU nurse was grinding her teeth.

"I am a nurse," she retorted. "I am not a gopher."

"You are a nurse," the supervisor yelled, "and you are whatever you have to be to try to save lives!"

The ICU nurse started crying and the patient coded.

"Go sit down until we can stabilize this patient," the supervisor ordered.

The nurse apologized to me for her behavior. She was written up and put on probation for that morning's events—at least that's what I heard through the grapevine— but she was never rude to anyone after that morning.

What the supervisor said was true for anyone in the healthcare industry. It's not my job to mop up a spill, but if I have to do that to avoid a patient or staff injury, I'll do it. I'm not a mother, but I've held a man's son while he was saying goodbye to his deceased wife.

The patient in question didn't die. She did have a heart attack, and she was placed on ICU for a week. When doctors questioned her, she said the last thing she remembered was thinking she had to go find her dog—the one that had died 20 years before her middle of the night journey. Somewhere along the way, the patient lost her slippers and her walker.

<u>Sweet Little Lies</u>

Four of the stories you read were pieces of fiction. Here are the answers, along with a commentary blurb for each one:

1.) Timber

I'll probably never get lucky enough to see a video of how a patient sustained his or her injury. I got the idea from watching a guy in the waiting room nod off and almost fall out of a chair.

2.) Firsthand Account

Last year, I was on my way to work when I saw a man in a pickup weave between the railroad arms. The train was probably about a foot from hitting the truck's bed. It made me think of how someone would react to seeing something like that and realizing the person lived.

3.) 32 Teeth Discount

If this ever happened at the hospital, I haven't heard about it. I forgot to thaw the chicken, so I had to stop by a grocery store really quick to grab dinner for work. While I was trying to decide what I wanted, I saw a woman (very clearly on drugs) walking around, eating from a deli box of fried chicken pieces. We arrived to separate checkout lines at the same time. As I was paying for my TV dinner, the woman was arguing with the cashier, saying she shouldn't have to pay for a full box of chicken because there was only one piece in it. I don't know what happened...I was running late.

4.) She's Got a Feelin'

Just kidding! This really happened.

4.) A (Made Up) Family Affair

While we did have a child purposely punch through a window (unlike the story's accident) and have to go to surgery, we've still never had a stranger come in and claim to be a patient's relative. But now that I've said that, I'm sure we will.

Sign from an MVA

While some of these stories contain details of patients doing stupid things to wind up in the ER with terrible injuries, sometimes it takes doing something ordinary to end up with a wild tale to tell friends.

After an ice storm one night, MVA victims started flooding in, mostly via ambulance. For the most part, the patients presented with fairly minor injuries: superficial lacerations, maybe a fractured bone here or there. But nobody came in with life-threatening injuries or had to be transferred out, so while it was busy, our energy wasn't getting sucked away like it does when one horrific injury comes over.

The ambulance radio went off for the ninth time in an hour and a half. Before dispatch started talking, we were taking bets on what would be called over. We all agreed it would be another MVA, and it was. But none of us won the pot (a 10-minute break and a candy bar) on the injury.

When he arrived, our newest patient—and elderly man— was covered in blood from his head to his mid-abdominal region. He was moaning and crying. I couldn't see too much of him, and what I could see passed by in a blur.

I went to the front to meet his wife. She was bruised around her eyes and blood stained her white blouse. She was also crying.

"Is he going to live?" were her first words.

I couldn't answer that, and I tried to take the woman's mind off of her husband's condition by asking her registration questions. Before I could finish the process, a nurse came to the front and asked the wife to come back immediately. The patient had lost consciousness and the doctor had questions regarding the man's medical and medicinal history.

I took what paperwork I had to the back and realized patients who'd been in rooms before the man arrived were all left alone in their rooms. Every nurse available hurried around the elderly man's room. One of the overnight doctors was speaking to the man's wife, blocking her view from the room. He was jotting the woman's replies to his questions down on a small steno notepad.

"It's really that bad?" I asked the unit clerk.

He nodded. "He's on blood thinner, and the accident was pretty bad. He's losing a lot of blood and they don't know if they can stop it."

"Did he just hit his head?"

The unit clerk shook his. "Before he passed out, he said he was in the passenger seat, with his cane between his legs. I guess they hit a patch of ice, and when they rolled, the cane flew up and scalped him. And then his head went through the passenger window. I guess he has a pretty big chunk of his skull detached. It sounds pretty bad."

It did sound pretty bad.

The ER doctor speaking to the wife guided her through the ER and asked her to speak to a counselor in the consult room.

That's never a good place to be in this hospital. It's similar to my religious questioning...if you get sent to the consult room, we know you are in need of isolation or protection, in a case such as an abusive relationship and you need to be out of sight in the instance that your abuser should walk in; or you're in there because your family member is dying.

Once the counselor spoke with the wife, the man's spouse decided she did wish to see her husband, despite the severity of his injuries. She said she would never be able to forgive herself if she didn't say goodbye, even if the image of his injuries stayed in her mind for the rest of her life.

Surprisingly, to me anyway, the patient lived for more than a year following the accident. He was transferred from our hospital to a trauma center several hours away, where he underwent surgery to reconstruct the missing portion of his skull and treat his scalping.

We all saw the patient and his wife a few months after the accident. Though scarred and still weak, the patient was in good spirits, and his wife spent half an hour crying and hugging the nurses and doctors. We learned the couple had been together since their teen years, and the night they presented to the ER for his injuries was their 75th anniversary. They took it as a sign that they really did belong together.

From a chart...

"Pt presents today with cc that she her shortness of breath is interfering with her ability to smoke her cigarettes."

My Wild Night AKA: Last Night AKA: Please Don't Make Me Go Back

The last shift of my week-long stretch is rarely slow. I think the universe knows how much I want to have a slow night, so instead, it throws every possible curve ball my direction to make me better appreciate my days off. Or maybe some higher power just likes pointing at me and saying, "Ha!"

Within 10 minutes of my evening-shift coworker walking out the door and leaving me up front all alone, five patients walked in, and the police scanner went off twice, alerting us of three patients en route due to an MVA with two older patients with suspected serious injuries, as well as a drunk driver with a suspected broken collarbone.

To top it all off, all five of the ambulatory patients were rude and impatient. None of them could understand why they weren't taken straight back for their superficial complaints, despite my explanation that the back was still full of rather serious complaints.

So, after 20 minutes of being alone at the

registration desk, the top of my Tracking Board was almost full and I couldn't see where the bottom part ended.

Family poured in for the elderly MVA patients, and EMS came out to get two of the members for each room, as the patients were anxious and panicking. Well, I guess the drunk driver of the MVA was being wheeled into a room at the same time as the family members were going back, and the next thing I knew, I heard EMTs, nurses, the family members, and an unidentified voice (later ID'd as the drunk driver) screaming. Security ran from the lobby to the back corridor. The elderly patients' family members were assaulting the drunk driver while he was still on the gurney.

What a mess already.

"Why were those people called back when they were here two seconds, yet I've been waiting twenty minutes?" demanded a patient from the waiting room.

"They were family members for another patient," I explained. "They weren't patients."

"I don't care who they are," the woman spit at me. "I want to know why they were taken back before me. You seem to have enough people free to come get other people, but you don't have enough people to take me back? Please."

I kind of stared at her. "Um, the guy that came out for those people doesn't even work here. And they were taken back because the patients in the back are facing serious injuries."

"You don't know I'm not."

I looked at the Tracking Board to remember why the woman was there. Oh, yeah...Burning with urination.

"We'll get you back as soon as we can," I sternly responded.

The woman cussed a little bit and then even more when security escorted the first members of the elderly patients' family out and switched out for two much calmer members.

I sat down and put my head in my hands.

Then the cops were on the police scanner.

"A pedestrian just flagged me down and said there's a subject passed out in the intersection of Road and Street. The subject is said to have vomit on his shirt and urinated. The pedestrian didn't have a way to notify EMS. I'm a few blocks away, so I'll check it out."

"Clear," the dispatcher replied.

Great.

I already knew we were about to get another patient. And it was Sunday night, so I was certain I'd see the police a few more times that night. For some reason, Sunday nights are when we see the most drug and alcohol-related patients.

"Dispatch, notify EMS that we need an ambulance at the intersection of Road and Street. Subject is a male, no ID. Subject is covered in vomit and urine."

I knew that wasn't all.

The temperatures in this part of Ohio dropped from high 60s to negative wind-chill within a matter of days, and the NWS released a warning that temperatures were dangerously low, with the chance of frostbite occurring within 30 minutes of being outside unprotected.

Static came across the radio, and I knew it was coming.

"Subject feels ice cold. Pulse feels about 40. He's displaying signs of frostbite on his fingers, nose, and ears. There are no witnesses to say how long subject has been unconscious."

I looked at the Tracking Board again. Four out of the 10 patients in back were being admitted, one was being discharged, and the rest were still up in the air.

And then the bed availability and the status of the ER was changed to red: nobody goes in, and nobody goes out. Either something was going dreadfully wrong in the back, or the nurses were preparing for the unconscious (and probably drunk) male.

It turned out to be both situations.

The drunk driver from the MVA started seizing, while the wife from the MVA exhibited stroke symptoms. Two techs were left to set up another trauma room for the incoming frostbite patient.

And then same woman from earlier came to the desk.

"This is getting ridiculous. I've been waiting for twenty-five minutes. You do know this is the emergency room, right?"

I wanted to say, "I do, but you apparently don't."

"What if this was a real emergency?" the woman

asked.

"Why don't you come back when you're really having one and let's see how it goes," I almost said.

But I didn't because I'm trying to get right with God and I don't think I'd be able to get Wi-Fi while living in a tent city after getting fired.

"Ma'am," I said calmly, "there are some pretty serious things going on in the back right now. The doctors have made the call to lock down the back part, which means new patients won't be brought back unless they're actively dying."

The woman cussed at me again. Instead of sitting down, she walked in circles around the lobby, going between waiting at the desk and staring out the window.

"I find it funny," she noted, "that you say it's *so* busy, yet the parking lot isn't even half full."

I rolled my eyes behind her back and ignored her.

An ambulance flew down the road with its lights and sirens blaring. Rather than pull in the bay, the ambulance raced through the parking lot and stopped in front of the ER. That doesn't happen here unless they can't wait for the bay doors to open.

This patient was dying.

As EMS scrambled to remove the patient from the back of the ambulance, I thought the complaining woman would go sit down, but she didn't. She just stood in front of the door and watched.

"Move!" one of the EMTs screamed at the lady as two medics ran a gurney through the foyer and toward the double doors I opened.

"Don't you dare talk to me that way," the woman retorted. "If I want to stand here, I'm going to—."

"Get out of the way now," the other medic ordered.

He didn't stop pushing the gurney. Neither of the men seemed to care that they ran into the woman with the end of the stretcher. They were focused on the frostbite patient...who was in cardiac arrest and foaming at the mouth.

Even though the woman saw the patient, she couldn't think of anyone but herself.

And that, folks, if you don't work in the healthcare industry, is probably the hardest point to get across to those in other industries. One would think humans would encompass some sense of compassion or decency or tolerance or patience in the ER—especially when hearing or seeing someone in a far worse condition—but most don't. People, these types are more prevalent in society than I ever imagined. They wouldn't care if you walked in with your leg hanging off or with half of your brain in the palm of your hand; they'd still demand to be seen before you.

"This is the worst hospital I've ever been to," the woman fumed. "This is ridiculous. I've been here a long time already, and nobody has even checked on me or offered me a drink or anything."

"You've been to a hospital where people offer you a drink?" I questioned.

I should have kept my mouth shut, but it just kind of fell out.

"You must go to those spa hospitals or something,

because every hospital I've ever been to has had at least a three-hour waiting time for the ER and patients weren't supposed to eat or drink until their test results came back. Maybe you should go back to that hospital. It sounds out of this world."

The woman shook her head. "Congratulations. You've just lost a customer. I'm going to tell everyone on Facebook about how crappy this place is, and I'll be sure to use your name."

And I was thinking, 'She knows my name?'

"Goodbye, Jane Doe," she said to me, nodding to my coworker's nameplate on the counter top.

I remembered I never removed the nameplate and giggled as the woman walked out the doors.

You know, I thought that was over, but I was so wrong.

The agitated woman didn't walk off to her car. Instead, she approached the parked ambulance and...no joke...she began swinging at the side mirrors with her big ole' (what looked expensive) handbag.

I knew security was busy, and I knew they wouldn't want to even touch down on this, so I did the only thing I knew to do: I called 911.

"What's your emergency?"

I identified myself and tried to explain myself coherently, but I blurted out, "This crazy woman is beating the crap out of an ambulance because she wasn't seen fast enough."

Dispatch started to place a call out to available units, but she didn't have to follow through. Three squad cars, two attached to the MVA from earlier and one there to check on the status of the frostbitten patient, noticed the woman's actions and surrounded her.

As officers tried to calm the woman down, EMS emerged from the back and saw the commotion.

"What is this nut doing to our ride?" one shouted. "We weren't even back there that long. What did we do to her?"

I couldn't hear what was happening outside, but as I glanced between the security monitors and the glass doors, I gathered the officers were trying to get the woman to stop her destructive behavior.

Like I said earlier...

I've never been in the situation, but if a police officer ever tells me to stop, I'm going to stop.

When multiple tired, cold, and busy officers tell me to stop, I'm going to stop even faster.

And if a cop ever opens his squad car door and brings out a K9 Unit, I'm going to stop, put my hands up, and try not to move even half a centimeter.

This woman, though...phew. She didn't stop. She didn't stop even faster. And she certainly didn't stop, put her hands up, or try not to move even half a centimeter.

Up until this point, I'd never seen a K9 unit in action, besides some public demonstration at a park to show how disciplined the dogs were.

This beautiful, slender German Shepherd with erect ears and a cold glare stood at attention, awaiting the order.

I watched the canine's handler. The man's lips moved ever-so-slightly, and the dog was off.

EMS was going wild. They'd apparently never seen the K9 unit in action, either.

I glanced over to the waiting room, and I swear, every last person stood with their noses pressed against the windows.

When I looked back outside, the police dog was dangling from the woman's forearm. Even then, she continued to move around and yell. She refused to drop her handbag and swatted at the dog's head.

I'm pretty sure we were all rooting for the dog.

The phone rang.

"Registration," I said, answering blindly.

"What the heck is going on out front?" asked the charge nurse.

I was so wrapped up in trying to watch the scene that I forgot to answer.

"Hello?"

"This woman broke the ambulance mirrors so I called 911, and now the K9 is attacking her."

"What?!"

The line went dead, but I was too mesmerized to hang up, so I just stood there in awe with my mouth hanging open and the phone piece still pressed against my ear.

Our charge nurse hurried up front and stood next to the EMTs.

The crazy woman was brought down by two officers and cuffed, while the K9 stood over her.

And, because the woman sustained bites from the K9 unit, she was brought back inside to be re-registered as a jail clearance. She was taken straight to the back, too, which I'm sure really ticked her off even more.

She was taken off to jail for battery against an officer (swatting at the dog), damaging property, disturbing the peace, and—my favorite, maybe—possession of meth and drug paraphernalia.

Things calmed down a few hours after the dog incident. Our MVA patients—all three—were transferred to other hospitals by back-to-back helicopters. The frostbitten patient came to and confessed to taking bath salts and drinking. I guess he passed out as he was walking home from a party. He estimated he left the party around 10 and wasn't picked up until roughly around 12:30. In the end, he lost two toes and part of a finger due to frostbite.

I have to say, especially since this was so recent, this was the craziest night I've ever experienced in the ER. I applaud inner-city ER employees for putting up with this kind of madness on a daily basis. Hats off to you.

Two grown men were brought in by separate officers for medical clearance. The men had been in a physical altercation.

As I registered the two, I learned the fight was a little more than getting drunk and fighting at a bar over a woman.

The two men, friends for years, had a tad bit much to drink, started playing Mario Kart, and ended their night by fist fighting over one man's repetitive use of tossing shells from his vehicle and pushing the other man's car off the edge of the racetrack multiple times.

In the one guy's defense, that is a jerk-move.

Both men were taken to jail for the night.

No word on what happened when they were released.

I guess there's a new study going on, where feces from donors with a certain genetic makeup are being turned into pills that can boost a person's immune system. To be honest, I haven't read much into this because the thought is kind of nasty.

We had a patient come in and confess to consuming his feces. He said something about it was 'evolution' or something equally weird to rationalize his habit.

He was eventually admitted to mental health.

Sugar Cookie Fight

One of my favorite stories from work happened a few years ago, when a teenager was brought in by police officers and approached the registration desk in tears.

"Is this a drug screen or a medical clearance?"

The cop shook his head and smirked. "Neither. Not yet, anyway. We're just going to send this gentleman here to the waiting room, and I need to go back for the ambulance that's about to arrive. If this wise guy decides to leave, please remind him there's an armed officer outside."

Hmm.

"Okay," I shrugged.

The officer told the crying teen to take a seat and wait for results. I had no idea what was going on.

I was called to the back to gather some information from the ambulance patient, another teen. His eyes were just as bloodshot as his friend's, and when he wasn't looking at me, he was vomiting.

"What happened here?" I asked the cop.

151

He laughed.

"These two geniuses decided to sniff model car glue and then have a wrestling match on the one kid's trampoline."

I crinkled my eyebrows.

It turns out, these two high teenagers decided to take their wrestling match to another level. They didn't want to hit each other with their fists, so they raided the one kid's kitchen for cookie sheets and thin pizza pans. Then, the two returned to the trampoline, where they took turns hitting each other with the pans.

From what I understood, the kid in the waiting room hit his friend upside the head with a cookie sheet hard enough to bend the pan in half. His friend was stunned by the hit, staggered backward, caught his ankle between the trampoline and the metal spring, and then fell off the trampoline, where he hit his head on the ground.

Because the first kid was high, he wasn't thinking all that clearly. He thought he killed his friend, so he dialed 911 to confess a murder.

When the police and EMTs arrived, they could see the other teen was simply unconscious, but they went along and played with the other kid, saying they were going to charge him with first degree murder and make sure he never saw the outside world again.

Nurses wrapped up the patient's sprained ankle and kept him until he came down from his high, while cops sat with the other kid until he was sober, too.

The officers agreed that the boys' embarrassment and fear was enough of a punishment, along with the fact that one of the boys' parents were ex-military and would add a suitable punishment of their own choosing.

One night, we could tell one of the medic teams and dispatch weren't getting along.

Call after call, we heard, "Medic 7, respond."

Even when there would be a delay for the patient, even when a closer team would respond, dispatch assigned the same team.

After about four hours of this, we couldn't take it anymore.

"Medic 7, respond."

My coworker faked a cry and yelled, "Leave Medic 7 alone!"

We get a lot of calls about the condition of the roads during winter.

I've started answering them by our MVA counts.

Most callers decide they 'don't really need to go out, then.'

A lot of people don't seem to know this, and I didn't either, until I started working at the hospital.

Nursing homes don't always call family members when a patient is transported to the ER, especially if the patient is brought in for a fall or an injury that could prove the facility has been neglectful in care.

One night, my coworker's mother was brought in via ambulance. When I saw my coworker walking around, laughing, I asked if she knew her mom was in the back.

She was the primary contact, but nobody called her because they didn't want the patient's family to know they had left the patient on a potty chair for hours and forgot about her.

"On a scale from 1 to 10, how would you rate your pain?"

"15."

We should be allowed to give out pamphlets that show the numbers from 1-35 on a chronological line.

I Take it Back

I've touched down on this before, but let me go ahead and explain our visiting procedures after seven pm to explain the story.

At seven, all entrances to the hospital lock, except for the ER doors. Visitors may exit from any door in the hospital, but to get back inside, they must enter through the emergency room. If a visitor wishes to visit a floor after open visiting hours, he or she must stop at the registration desk and speak with security. A security guard then asks for the visitor's ID, makes a copy, calls the floor for permission to send up a visitor, writes out a pass that is good for 12 hours, and then the security guard escorts the visitor through several badge-through doors until they reach the elevators. It's a process set in place for safety reasons above all, and it's usually hit or miss if someone's going to be mad about the process.

There are times people get snobby about the procedure, stating they have been visiting all day long and weren't told they'd have to get a pass, so that means they shouldn't have to. Some people say they shouldn't have to get a pass because it's a waste of time. People become angry when the guards have to ask for ID or when the guards call upstairs to make sure visitors are allowed.

In some instances, I can certainly understand visitors' grievances. Security will often skip the passes if the visitor needs to go to the hospice floor, or if they come in and say a family member just died.

Other times, however, I have been grateful that security's process meant they had to check with the floor. In several instances, on the OB floor especially, visitors have been denied due to family disputes or domestic violence or a huge mess of other excuses. When the visitors were told no, they all became loud and aggressive. I can only imagine what would have happened if the visitors actually made it to the floor and were dismissed.

Now that you know the process, you'll know why the man at the desk was waiting for security to give him back his ID.

What you wouldn't know—and what we didn't know—was why the mad was nervously shuffling his feet and tapping his fingertips on the counter.

"Are you okay?" I asked.

He sucked on his lips. "No. No, I don't think I am. I feel kind of lightheaded."

"Do you want to be seen?"

He shook his head. "No."

The man leaned over the counter and asked me, "Are they checking for warrants?"

I laughed, said no, and explained the security process.

The man seemed relieved, and I kept typing away in a chart.

Then curiosity got the best of me.

"Why would you ask that? Do you have a warrant out?"

The man laughed. "No. I just get nervous. I just got out of jail not too long ago because I failed to appear at my case for not paying rent. So now I'm paranoid."

I nodded. "Okay. Well, nobody's checking for warrants, so you should be okay."

The man still appeared nervous, but I didn't say anything else.

Security came back to the desk, wrote out a pass, and escorted the visitor upstairs.

While he was gone, a cop walked out from the back, after grabbing the results from a drug screening earlier. He walked by the desk, but then walked backwards and looked down at the copy of the driver's license security had just made.

"Where'd you get this?" he asked me.

"Oh," I said, "security makes copies of IDs before taking visitors up to floors."

"He's here now?" the cop asked.

I nodded and leaned over to check the carbon copy of the pass book. "It looks like he went up to the third floor."

The officer immediately snatched the radio attached

to his shoulder.

"Dispatch, this is Officer [Whatever] and I need another unit dispatched to [our hospital]. I've located [the visitor's name]."

Dispatch came over the radio to clear the request and then the woman started calling in another unit.

"Be advised this subject is considered armed and dangerous unless determined otherwise. Subject is wanted for armed robbery."

She went on to list a slew of other charges against the visitor, and I honestly was a bit surprised because I figured if the man had any warrants, they wouldn't be for all the things the dispatcher just listed off.

The guard who walked the patient up didn't have any idea that anything was wrong when he saw the officer standing by the registration desk. We have EMS, police, firefighters, and all kinds of other departments stop by the desk to chat about how the night's going, so nothing was out of the ordinary.

"I'm going to need you to notify that floor to get as far away from that subject as possible, without raising concern," the officer told the guard.

In total, four armed officers went up to the floor and arrested the man without incident. He surrendered himself peacefully to the officers and stated he didn't want to further upset his mother, whom he was visiting after her surgery.

<u>Can't Judge If I Do It, Too</u>

I was kinda-sorta a patient one night, unofficially, due to getting a little too wild at home.

My rental place has wood floors in the living room and bedroom. To get to the bedroom, I have to take a step down.

Well, I was getting a bit too carried away with dancing to the classics, wearing a new pair of those super-soft socks, when I thought it would be a fantastic idea to try that *Risky Business* thing. I've actually never seen that movie, but I know the part where he slides through the room. The only difference here was that I had pants on. Well, I guess that wasn't the only difference.

When *I* tried this, I not only fell and busted my butt, but I also went to stand up, tripped over the long ends of my pajama pants, and fell face-forward over that drop-off. The only move my dog made from the couch was to look at me like I was stupid, and I can't exactly say he was wrong at that point.

I went in to see a nurse on my night off, and yes, I

had a swollen nose, bruises on my tailbone, and two black eyes.

One of the doctors took a quick look at me and determined my nose wasn't broken, just cracked on the bridge.

I tried to be polite when I asked my coworker for a shot of Dilaudid and a meal tray.

Made in the USA
Middletown, DE
30 December 2018